BE F*#%ING AMAZING!

70 Healing Insights to Live Your Full Life

Also By Deborah Lucero
Online Courses

Healing Insights 70-Day Course
The 5-Step Process For Fibromyalgia Relief

Monthly Subscription Plan

The Wellness Plan
Please Visit:
Deborah's website: www.liveyourfulllife.com

BE F*#%ING AMAZING!

70 Healing Insights to Live Your Full Life

DEBORAH LUCERO

BALBOA.
PRESS

A DIVISION OF HAY HOUSE

Balboa Press books may be ordered through booksellers or by contacting:

Balboa Press
A Division of Hay House
1663 Liberty Drive
Bloomington, IN 47403
www.balboapress.com
1 (877) 407-4847

Cover and Interior Images Courtesy of Alex (TRI) Lucero and Ezekiel L. Lucero

ISBN: 978-1-9822-0889-9 (sc)
ISBN: 978-1-9822-0888-2 (e)

Library of Congress Control Number: 2018908502

Print information available on the last page.

Balboa Press rev. date: 10/23/2018

Editor credit: Michelle Josette

Table of Contents

Acknowledgments

I am grateful to many incredible people for the opportunity to write this book! I want to personally thank my loving family, caring medical team, and many generous personal growth and self-development mentors. My supportive husband, Alex, your kind words and encouragement helped me achieve my goals. My oldest son, Alex (aka "TRI"), you are my greatest mentor. Thank you for believing in me! My youngest son, Ezekiel, you are my hero! Thank you for teaching me to never give up. I love you all!

A special thank-you to my caring medical team. Thank you all for being in the right profession. I'm so thankful for the fantastic medical care that you all provide! Your extra effort to make a difference in the lives of your patients is appreciated.

I want to express my gratitude for the generosity of all the personal growth and self-development mentors. Most of you have never met me, however, the goodwill and love that you spread through your message is a blessing! I am fortunate for all the wisdom I have gained.

The following individuals have been a huge factor in helping me access my ability to heal.

To Nicole Englert at Arizona Allergy & Asthma Institute. Thank you for helping me to find a way to feel better. Thank you for sharing alternative treatments which helped me so much. Self-care did make a drastic difference in my life. Thank you for seeing the hope in me and not being afraid to express yourself! I'm glad you continue to help many others through the AAA Alliance Program. Keep spreading the word of hope.

To Dr. Mark Hyman at http://drhyman.com/. Thank you for developing *The Blood Sugar Solution 10-Day Detox Diet*. I completed your detox diet under the supervision of an allergist physician assistant, back in September 2014. Thank you for sharing so much insight with others! I sincerely wish you health and happiness.

To Nick Ortner at www.thetappingsolution.com. Thank you for helping me find a way to cope with all the emotions that I had bottled up for decades. I am grateful for you helping me realize, "I Am Enough!" Thank you for not being afraid to reach your full potential.

To my 'Tapping group,' Debra, Ashley, and Betty. Thank you, ladies, for participating in my pilot program for the Healing Insights 70-Day Course. I enjoyed our time each day as we 'Tapped,' chatted, and healed!

I am so grateful to everyone for helping me learn how to create a space to heal my mind, body, soul, and spirit.

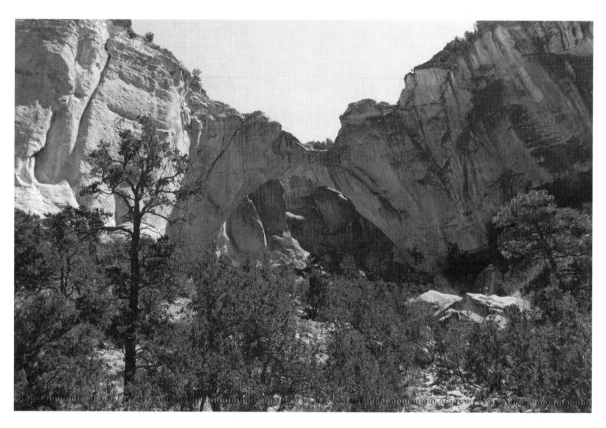

"The eyes are the window to your soul."
~William Shakespeare~

How (and Why) This Book Can Improve Your Life Mind, Body, Soul & Spirit Forever

What you will learn in this book not only gives you the steps to nurture your mind, body, soul, and spirit but also the ability to be successful. The techniques will show you how to detox, release emotion, create a positive mindset, reprogram your mind, and incorporate exercise/physical activity to heal your mind, body, soul, and spirit. Once you learn to access the miraculous healing power of your mind, you will be inspired to create the life you deserve.

Do You Know Why?

Why do you feel stuck and confused? Ever felt like you knew things were bound to get better, but you just couldn't turn things around? Ever wonder how other people can find a way to push through life's struggles? How do they achieve health, wealth, love, and happiness even after horrible circumstances? Trying to figure out how to hold on long enough? How to shift the tide, so to speak? Have you tried an alternative treatment, home remedies, taken a self-development course, or enrolled in counseling; but resolution seemed to escape you? Did you pull through these challenging situations, but ended up feeling incomplete or dissatisfied? Why is the entire thought of improving your life absolutely exhausting? Is there an answer to these questions that lies within the power of the mind? Yes. There absolutely is!

Why I Wrote This Book

This book was written to answer the questions in the section above and to give you the steps to live your full life. My goal was to explain the power of the mind as clearly as possible based on the healing insights I gained from immersing myself in this journey of personal growth and self-development. I used the many books, self-development courses, webinars, videos, and email newsletters to create a new mindset, to reprogram my mind, to take a leap of faith and believe in myself, to access the power of the mind. I chose to love and honor my mind, body, soul, and spirit! I would have never imagined that my journey through hell would eventually lead me to understand how I could create 'heaven on Earth.'

Master this knowledge of how the brain and body work and apply it to your own life. When you do, the steps become effortless. I feel empowered knowing the techniques I teach you will change your life forever! I am blessed to offer you this wisdom so you can live your full life. I hope you understand how vital these insights are for your healing, your enjoyment of life, and to achieve your full potential. Let these healing insights work amazing wonders in your body and in your life. Indulge in the power of the mind to heal your mind, body, soul, and spirit. Recognize that your situation, no matter how difficult it is right now, can and will get better. You *can* achieve health, wealth, love, and happiness!

Accessing the Power of The Mind

The most compelling evidence of the power of the mind is that of one's healing.

I went from being drugged up, asleep on my couch, taking 18 prescription medications a day to only taking all-natural vitamins and supplements. I was diagnosed with fibromyalgia and several other related medical conditions, in July of 2013. I was in so much pain that my prescriptions included narcotics like hydrocodone, morphine, and gabapentin.

I had excruciating pain in every joint, my jaw and ear hurt so bad from a temporomandibular joint (TMJ) disorder. I was having headaches and migraines that made me bedridden. I had muscle spasms so intense it felt like I had a heart attack. My intestinal health was a mess. I was only able to use the restroom once or maybe twice a week. My bladder was on fire. It felt like someone had a match over my genital area. My pelvic floor was spasming out of control. I had pain in my pelvic area and bladder for up to two days after intimacy with my husband. I developed gastritis which made me have a burning sensation that started in my stomach and went up to my throat and inside both of my nostrils. My entire body felt like I was in hell! I was inflamed, I was burning; I was in pain.

So how did I stop taking 18 prescription medications that I desperately needed for several different diagnoses to only taking natural vitamins and supplements?

I want to share with you not only the pain and the misery from the struggles that I faced and conquered, but also the hope, the healing, and the peace that you can have using the techniques I learned during the most challenging time in my life. I have created a five-step process to help you heal. The 5-Step Process includes Detox, Releasing Emotion, Mindset, Reprogramming Your Mind, and Exercise/Physical Activity.

All five of these steps are crucial in healing the mind, body, soul, and spirit. Western medicine has forgotten that you are a whole person. Your mind, body, soul, or spirit cannot be separated. You are all, and that is why this process includes techniques to heal each of these areas. I invite you to participate in my proven 5-Step Process to take back your health, to take control of your life, to find relief today!

Thoughts Transform When You Surrender

You can't just have a positive thought to access the power of the mind. You must have a positive thought while experiencing higher-level emotions such as gratitude, joy, acceptance, service, and love. Once you realize that this is the secret, you can give your conscious mind the blueprint it needs so the subconscious mind can carry out the plan to your benefit.

I realized that there are three essential parts. Your thoughts have to matter to send out positive energy. You have to make your thoughts and emotions match by surrendering your mind, body, soul, and spirit. You must take action to attract positive effects back to you!

Learn these simple steps to access the power of the mind. Re-read this book over and over again until you master this skill. Give yourself the opportunity to see the endless possibilities! Use this book to guide you through the process so you can realize your full potential to attain health, wealth, love, and happiness!

Everybody Surrenders

Do you know how to surrender completely?

The problem with completely surrendering is related to the stress response cycle. So many of us are overwhelmed by stress daily. Just thinking about stressful situations makes your mind and body believe it has to protect you. In response to this perceived threat, stress hormones are released, an immediate physiological response. Stress keeps you from being able to think clearly, to problem-solve, and to be resourceful. It damages your overall well-being when you are stuck in it for an extended period of time. The stress response cycle keeps you trapped. You are unable to comprehend, use your mind, intelligence, compassion, kindness, or better judgment. It keeps you from healing, which prevents you from being able to surrender completely.

In my book, I speak of healing. Healing doesn't just mean physical health. It means healing your mind, body, soul, and spirit. Emotional and spiritual health is just as important as physical health. It is of great significance that you understand to live a full life you must heal your mind, body, soul, and spirit!

I was miserable even before my health crashed. Like most people, I was tired of feeling stuck, limited, and disgusted. I felt as if I had done everything right, but I hadn't achieved health, wealth, love, or happiness. What was I missing? I discovered that you must totally surrender while you embrace your body to reach total health, forgive your mind to accomplish endless wealth, love your soul to achieve true love, and honor your spirit to create pure happiness.

People stuck in the stress response cycle can't access the power of the mind. For this reason, they need a simple step-by-step process to follow, along with a helping hand. My proven 5-Step Process is the steady guidance they need to heal their mind, body, soul, and spirit!

Distinct Features of This Book

There are five distinct features of this book.

1. Real-Life Techniques in Simple Terms

The real-life techniques are explained in simple terms for you to easily apply to your daily life and to every level of your being.

2. My Proven 5-Step Process

I have taught this simple step-by-step process in my Healing Insights 70-Day Course and The 5-Step Process For Fibromyalgia Relief course. It is followed by The Wellness Plan, a monthly subscription plan to maintain lasting change, to apply the five steps to daily life.

3. 70 Healing Insights

I created 70 Healing Insights for the Healing Insights 70-Day Course based on the research and information below. It was my goal to design a self-development course that provides enough content to give you the time to create new habits in your life. This course also deepens the concepts of my proven 5-Step Process.

In Tai Lopez's *67 Steps*, he mentioned a study conducted by University College of London: "What we found was that it takes 66 days on average for people in our study to acquire a habit," said Professor Jane Wardle of University College London, who carried out the study with Dr. Phillippa Lally. https://www. huffingtonpost.com/james-clear/forming-new-habits_b_5104807.html

I realized that this concept of 66 days was backed by research. I wanted to not only give you the steps to heal your mind, body, soul, and spirit, but also the ability to be successful. What better way than to provide enough content to give you the time to create new habits in your life? I also thought, how can I make this work to deepen the concepts of The 5-Step Process? My favorite number has always been 7 and when I divided 70 by 5, I came up with 14 days for each step. I thought, perfect! Plus, my sign is Libra so having a balanced number made it seem like 70 days was meant to be!

4. Body, Mind, Soul, and Spirit

Everything I have always read related to spirituality refers to body, mind, and spirit. What about the soul? I thought, I guess the two are interchangeable, right? I began reading *Adventures of the Soul* by

James Van Praagh, where soul and spirit are defined so clearly. His explanation helped me understand the relationship between the two.

Here is an excerpt from his book: "I often think of Glinda, the Good Witch from the Wizard of Oz, when I contemplate the soul returning to Spirit. Remember the image of Glinda inside her bubble traveling up, up, and away? Think of Glinda as your soul and Spirit as the bubble as you make the journey home. The soul returns to Spirit, and just as the body is an expression of the soul, so too is the soul an expression of Spirit."

I have chosen to include the mind, body, soul, and spirit because we cannot be separated. We are a whole being.

5. All This Wisdom in One Spot

Plus, my proven 5-Step Process has captured all this wisdom in one spot! Don't spend hours searching for all this healing insight; it is right here for you to use it, right now! Don't have to waste your precious time. You can start applying these healing insights immediately to live the life you deserve. Matthew Syed, the author of *Bounce*, discovered that it takes 10,000 hours of practice to master a skill. Use your 10,000 hours to master The 5-Step Process to live your full life!

The distinct features of this book will help you reveal the answer to the question. "What is the 'one thing' I've been missing so I can achieve the life I deserve?"

You will find the reasons for this shared concern. You will learn precisely how to access the power of the mind. You will learn how to apply this process to improve all areas of your life.

What Are Your Beliefs?

It is not just the ability to access the power of the mind but the thoughts behind this dominant force that transform ideas into reality. 'You are the placebo' simply means that whatever you believe in will heal you. The definition of the 'placebo effect' is positive thoughts that generate positive effects.

Remember, you must not just think a thought; you must feel it, in every fiber of your being. You must observe that desire as if it has already taken place. You must send out that positive energy and surrender your mind, body, soul, and spirit completely. Only then are you capable of attracting all that your heart desires.

Your reality will become something that you can build just by thought!

Hope is Desire

Everyone desires health, wealth, love, and happiness. We have all been there—feeling stuck, limited, and disgusted. You may have tried keeping your New Year's resolution by signing up at the gym; or gone back to college to improve your skills for the workforce; enrolled in couple's counseling to make that special relationship work; or tried to be happy despite your situation, but still, health, wealth, love, and happiness have slipped through your fingers. Even though you did everything you were told and thought you knew what you needed to succeed, you don't feel successful or happy. Instead, you feel trapped and inadequate. Finally, discover that 'one thing' you've been missing, so you can attain health, wealth, love, and happiness!

By learning the techniques that worked for me, you will have everything you need to live your full life. If you take action, implementing my proven 5-Step Process will change your beliefs about the power of the mind, positive thoughts, and an abundant mindset. The key reason for this is because you will be inspired to honor your mind, body, soul, and spirit so you can allow yourself to heal. You will learn how to process and release recurring situations keeping you stuck. Once you eliminate these obstacles, you can use the power of the mind like never before to realize your full potential!

There is only one process of healing and that is faith. There is only one healing power, namely, your subconscious mind.

(Joseph Murphy)

The healing power of your subconscious mind existed in your spirit before you took on your physical form. Comprehend that you have two minds that operate as a team, your conscious and subconscious mind. Your conscious mind creates the plan (a thought), and your subconscious mind carries it out to turn it into a reality. This miraculous healing power will materialize the thoughts and beliefs of your spirit. That is why your thoughts matter! Whether you have a positive or negative thought, it will happen. Keep this in mind! I strongly advise you to follow the steps in this book to enhance your life, to improve your well-being, and to honestly be happy.

The only thing you have to do is think a positive thought and make your feelings match. These feelings are the connection between thoughts and actions that cause changes to take place starting in your body, then in your life and the world around you. When your body, mind, soul, and spirit are tuned in to your thoughts, feelings, and actions, your life will change. There are no limits to what you can accomplish with this knowledge. The question is not if it will work. It is proof of how it works!

You can create a space to heal. You can move forward in your life and create a new mindset, a mindset that belongs to you, a mindset free of false beliefs, a mindset free of doubt. It's your time. It's your life. The possibilities are endless! You must observe it so it can become a reality. You can attain it. You can live big! You have the potential to live the life you dreamed of when you were a child—that big life you envisioned when you were developing your character, your interests, and your goals. The most exciting part of creating The 5-Step Process is to share with you all these healing insights! To give you the matter-of-fact, concrete proof that you can create the life you deserve. You have to know how to maximize for a full life.

CHAPTER ONE

Step 1 Detox: Healing Insights 1–14

Detox your mind, body, soul, and spirit from thoughts, emotions, events, relationships, unhealthy food, old programs, false beliefs, and bad habits!

When I began this journey, I was allergic to more than 40 food items. I had lost about 30 pounds and felt miserable! I never learned proper nutrition as a child. My diet consisted of foods laced with sugar, fat, and salt. I was addicted to processed foods and ate fast food or unhealthy restaurant food at least five times per week.

What I was about to learn about detox would turn my world upside down. Or should I say right side up! What I share with you will help you understand how commercials, the food industry, and the bad habits you learn as a child shape your mindset. This misinformation becomes the beliefs and programs that your subconscious mind runs automatically every day of your life.

This chapter helps you realize that just as you become addicted to unhealthy food, you become addicted to thoughts, emotions, events, and relationships not serving you. This addiction is made stronger by chemicals released in your body as you think, feel, and react to your environment. Over time, your body becomes trapped in the stress response cycle which keeps you from the self-care your mind, body, soul, and spirit need to live your full life.

Healing Insight 1: I see the hope in you.

Nicole Englert, PA, Arizona Allergy & Asthma Institute

When I met the physician assistant (PA) at my allergist office I thought it was by chance. My allergist had called in sick the day of my appointment, and I was offered an appointment with his PA. I initially refused the offer. But something inside me said, "You feel miserable, maybe you should go." So, I called back and kept the appointment.

I just kept thinking, *Now I have to rehash everything to bring her up to speed since I have never seen her before. What a pain.* I still felt reluctant even as I sat in the waiting room. I am usually thorough in reporting symptoms and updates from other medical providers, but I wasn't feeling up to starting from square one that day.

Here is an excerpt from my symptom log.

9/14/14

9:00am—appt AZ Asthma & Allergy Institute-Reported to Nicole Englert, Physician Assistant (PA) (no change) /continue (con't) symptoms: Left (L) side cheek/nasal pressure, jaw/ear pain, colored mucus since last week in April, increased post-nasal drip/sore throat. Reminded PA that computerized axial tomography (CT) scan ruled out nasal fungus & nasal polyp, mild inflammation ethmoid sinus & no change with antibiotics (Baclofen, Levaquin). Discussed food sensitivities, tried most foods—exhibited symptoms with (w/) majority. PA recommended con't strict nasal hygiene regimen (humidifier—nighttime, nasal wash, saline spray, allergy meds, Flonase & decongestant) pro re nata (PRN—as needed), added syringe medications after nasal wash (if covered by insurance) & follow up (F/U) w/ ear, nose, throat (ENT) for sinus culture—recommended by ENT. PA suggested the following for general health: probiotic, fish oil, Dr. Hyman's *The Blood Sugar Solution 10-Day Detox Diet*, Raw Meal protein (cautioned to check ingredients due food sensitivities). PA provided AAA Alliance Program resources to improve gut health/overall well-being (UHCCP does not cover). F/U 10/02/14 1pm.

To my surprise, the PA had experienced many of the same medical conditions and symptoms I had. She had been out of work for over a year and had recently returned and started the AAA Alliance Program which was established to provide resources to patients with chronic conditions to improve their general health, gut health, and general well-being. Even though my insurance did not cover the cost for me to participate in the AAA Alliance Program, she gave me the resources I needed to get started.

When she showed me a two-inch fresh scar on her face near her ear from surgery due to TMJ disorder, I knew she knew my pain. She could relate and have compassion. She said, "I see the hope in you." To this day I get emotional when I relive this memory because I was at such a low place in my life at the time. I couldn't even see the hope in myself. This touched me on a deep level.

At the time, it hurt to do any and everything. I had pain in my jaw and ears from TMJ disorder, which led to headaches and migraines causing pain in my left jaw, ear, temple, and pain behind my left eye. I had pain in my neck from cervical sprain (whiplash) from a car accident I was in, the month of April 2014. I had a burning pain in my stomach, throat, sinus passages, and nostrils from gastritis and food allergies. My skin was extremely sensitive. Even scratching burned terribly; it was as if someone had raked a knife across my skin. I had weird, painful, burning sensations across my cheeks and arms.

I had such severe muscle spasms I felt like I had a heart attack! I had breast pain from dense breast tissue. I had chronic sciatica which was exacerbated in 2012 from all the sitting behind a desk and driving to and from work. I had pain in every joint. Although my internal organs were functioning, they were highly inflamed according to the rheumatologist who diagnosed me with central sensitivity syndrome with fibromyalgia in July 2013.

I had throbbing, pinching pain under my right-side rib cage because my liver enzyme levels were elevated. My gastroenterologist discovered it was from all the prescription medications I was taking. I had chronic constipation. I was so backed up that I only had a bowel movement maybe once or twice a week. My liver enzyme level of alanine aminotransferase (ALT) and serum glutamic pyruvic transaminase (SGPT) was 67 IU/L. The normal range is 0–32.

Comp. Metabolic Panel (14)

Test	Result	Flag	Unit	Limits	Lab
Glucose, Serum	82		mg/dL	65 - 99	PDLCA
BUN	15		mg/dL	6 - 24	PDLCA
Creatinine, Serum	0.49	L	mg/dL	0.57 - 1	PDLCA
eGFR If NonAfricn Am	120		mL/min/1.73	>59	PDLCA
eGFR If Africn Am	138		mL/min/1.73	>59	PDLCA
BUN/Creatinine Ratio	31	H		9 - 23	PDLCA
Sodium, Serum	140		mmol/L	134 - 144	PDLCA
Potassium, Serum	4.1		mmol/L	3.5 - 5.2	PDLCA
Chloride, Serum	100		mmol/L	97 - 108	PDLCA
Carbon Dioxide, Total	28		mmol/L	18 - 29	PDLCA
Calcium, Serum	9.7		mg/dL	8.7 - 10.2	PDLCA
Protein, Total, Serum	6.6		g/dL	6 - 8.5	PDLCA
Albumin, Serum	4.5		g/dL	3.5 - 5.5	PDLCA
Globulin, Total	2.1		g/dL	1.5 - 4.5	PDLCA
A/G Ratio	2.1			1.1 - 2.5	PDLCA
Bilirubin, Total	0.3		mg/dL	0 - 1.2	PDLCA
Alkaline Phosphatase, S	82		IU/L	39 - 117	PDLCA
AST (SGOT)	39		IU/L	0 - 40	PDLCA
ALT (SGPT)	67	H	IU/L	0 - 32	PDLCA

Lab results date collected 2/24/2015.

I had burning pain and pressure in my bladder from interstitial cystitis (a.k.a. bladder pain syndrome.) This condition makes you feel like you have a urinary tract infection (UTI) constantly. My ability to travel was restricted because the movement of just riding in a vehicle increased my bladder pain. I had pelvic floor spasms which gave me severe pain during intimacy. This pain lasted for up to two days due to spastic pelvic floor syndrome also known as pelvic floor tension myalgia. Sadly, I did not get this condition diagnosed until November 2014.

I struggled with anemia and severe vitamin D deficiency. My vitamin D level was 10.6 L. The normal range is between 30.01 and 100.0 ng/mL.

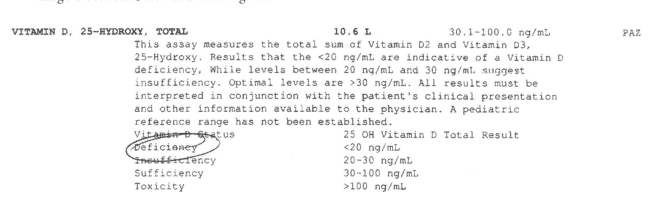

```
VITAMIN D, 25-HYDROXY, TOTAL            10.6 L           30.1-100.0 ng/mL           PAZ
              This assay measures the total sum of Vitamin D2 and Vitamin D3,
              25-Hydroxy. Results that the <20 ng/mL are indicative of a Vitamin D
              deficiency, While levels between 20 ng/mL and 30 ng/mL suggest
              insufficiency. Optimal levels are >30 ng/mL. All results must be
              interpreted in conjunction with the patient's clinical presentation
              and other information available to the physician. A pediatric
              reference range has not been established.
              Vitamin D Status            25 OH Vitamin D Total Result
              Deficiency                  <20 ng/mL
              Insufficiency               20-30 ng/mL
              Sufficiency                 30-100 ng/mL
              Toxicity                    >100 ng/mL
```

Lab results date collected 1/2/2013.

My allergist recommended I maintain a level in the high fifties due to allergies and asthma.

I also had to change positions at least every thirty minutes because I felt pain after fifteen to thirty minutes of sitting, standing, walking, or lying down. Yes, it hurt to sit, stand, walk, lie down, eat, sleep, pee, poop, and be intimate.

By the time I met the PA I wanted my life to be over. I cried while being intimate with my husband. I asked him to assist me in my death. I wanted to be dead. The only thing stopping me from committing suicide was that I believed I would be stuck in purgatory. I was absolutely miserable. I had to find a way to be done with feeling this pain and fatigue every day, even if it meant death. I went as far as researching the states that allowed doctor-assisted suicide. At the time, four states allowed it. I share this to give you an idea of how truly miserable, fed up, and wiped out I was.

The PA had my full attention when she said, "I see the hope in you!" I didn't think I had anything left inside me to fight back. But her statement truly inspired me to move! I followed her recommendations and started Dr. Hyman's *The Blood Sugar Solution 10-Day Detox Diet*. Even though it was designed to help people who were diabetic or obese, it had a section for skinny-fat people (people who are skinny but ill). I fit that profile perfectly! I tried probiotics and fish oil. I also tried the protein, but unfortunately, it did not agree with me due to food allergies. I was open to any and all suggestions because I knew one thing: I was sick and tired of being sick and tired!

Again, I tell my story to share with you the hope, the healing, and the peace. Please know you can find a way to feel better. There are alternative treatments out there. Self-care does make a difference. I will show you how, starting with a tapping meditation for hope, healing, and peace at hope.liveyourfulllife. com. Please join me so you can create a space for your body, mind, soul, and spirit to heal.

Please know, I am with you on this journey. I know it is a difficult one. But I am here to help you; I am here to guide you. Thank you again for joining me!

Healing Insight 2: I can be healthy!

The Blood Sugar Solution 10-Day Detox Diet, Dr. Mark Hyman

It wasn't until I started to follow Dr. Mark Hyman that I made a huge realization that I could actually be healthy. As I prepared to begin Dr. Mark Hyman's detox diet I listened to his audiobook, *The Blood Sugar Solution 10-Day Detox Diet*, reviewed the recipes, did my kitchen detox, and bought vitamins and supplements. My husband bought me a Ninja food processor as suggested by my allergist's PA. I was ready to go!

In addition, I explored Dr. Hyman's website. I signed up for his email list to receive newsletters, videos, and free online summits. That's when I first heard about functional medicine. *Functional medicine* simply means treating the cause of the problem rather than just the symptoms. Doing this can reverse symptoms and even medical conditions altogether. I thought, *Wow, I, actually have the ability to be healthy again!* I questioned how this could be possible with all my medical conditions. I discovered the ability to heal lies in being responsible and caring for yourself as a whole being!

I thought, *How can this be*? The doctors said there is no cure for fibromyalgia, interstitial cystitis (IC), or irritable bowel syndrome (IBS). I kept asking myself, "How can I be healthy again?" But I listened to

Dr. Hyman about how self-care, diet, exercise, lifestyle changes, vitamins/supplements, and improved sleep were all my responsibility according to the concept of functional medicine.

It blew my mind when I heard that only 5% of medical conditions are genetic. That means 95% of medical conditions are due to lifestyle factors. *OMG! How could this be?* I was taught diabetes, hypertension, obesity, cancer, heart disease, etc. were all genetic. I said, "What the H***!" My thought was, *Maybe I can be healthy?* I was confused, excited, and angry. But I was hopeful that I could take back my health, take control of my life, and find relief. Now more than ever I was ready to start the diet.

Remember, your thoughts cause feelings and your feelings cause changes in your body! A negative thought leads to a negative emotion like anger which makes your body release a hormone such as adrenaline. Then you feel angrier! A positive thought leads to a positive emotion like happiness which causes your body to release a hormone like dopamine. Then you feel happier! Can you see how this becomes a cycle? Don't you agree that a positive cycle is best?

Healing Insight 3: Know your triggers!

The Tapping Solution: A Revolutionary System for Stress-Free Living, Nick Ortner

This sounds simple, right? But it's not always as clear-cut as it seems. Sure, traffic jams, rushing to make dinner, and trying to make ends meet financially are all common triggers. But what about the subtle triggers of losing the battle to your symptoms, relying on others to pick up the slack, and trying to hold on to anything that resembles a normal life?

This healing insight was especially difficult for me because I am a perfectionist. If I can just maintain some level of control about the situation, I can survive. But with so many body parts screaming with never-ending pain, everything seemed to be a trigger! I hated not being able to control the aches and pains stealing my life. I felt as if my body, mind, soul, and spirit were being stripped away from me. I needed desperately to get a handle on the main triggers causing me to spin out of control!

But how? My finances were a joke, my body wouldn't stop hurting, and the stress I was continually experiencing was making me violent. I can only describe how I felt like being revved up! In February 2014, during two separate physical therapy sessions, my physical therapist noticed my tension. I sat at the edge of the chair. My shoulders were elevated, and I clenched my teeth. My therapist said, "Gee, you look like you're ready to jet!" On a different day, I sat at the edge of my chair with my hands clenched into fists so tight that my knuckles were white. My therapist said, "Sit back and relax."

In mid-October 2014, I received a newsletter from Dr. Mark Hyman. I had signed up on his website the month before while I was researching his 10-Day Detox Diet. The newsletter mentioned Emotional Freedom Techniques (tapping). The email provided a link to a free webinar offered by Nick Ortner at The Tapping Solution. The webinar was titled, *How to Create an Abundant Stress-Free Financial Future Faster Than You Ever Thought Possible.* According to Ortner, the secret was the technique of tapping! I figured, *What do I have to lose?* and registered for the webinar.

I convinced my husband to watch it with me during dinner that week. The webinar included hands-on activities to journal, answer questions, and Nick led us through a tapping meditation. Somehow, I felt better after participating in the tapping meditation. I hadn't felt calm for the last couple of years. I even felt safe which I didn't understand totally, although Nick Ortner explained the process of tapping in detail. Curious about the whole idea of tapping, I visited The Tapping Solution website.

Because I had been stuck in the stress response cycle for so long, I still felt on edge. Tapping wasn't working fast enough for me to deal with my ever-increasing aggression. I would wake up and feel as if my blood was boiling and my skin was crawling. I was so angry and disgusted because I could not help myself. I felt like I could lose control at any moment. I was impatient, rude, hateful, and mean with my family.

Despite the way I felt, I kept tapping. I had moments of calm and feelings of safety. But one day my husband commented, and I lost it! After returning from a chiropractor adjustment, I mentioned to my husband the chiropractor wanted to see me twice a month. My husband jokingly replied, "Who's going to pay for it?" Finances were a sensitive topic since I was not working at the time. Due to all the medical conditions, I was having difficulty managing. I reacted so poorly. I am ashamed of what happened.

I share this story only because the importance it plays in knowing your triggers and feeling safe. My anger and aggression came on so quickly. My head filled with blood. My face felt hot. My husband worked from home at the time and was seated at his computer desk. I formed fists and hit him on the back with all my might. I pounded on the wall in the hallway with such force, it caused some bladder leakage. At that moment, I heard my husband getting up from his chair and I ran into the bathroom and locked the door.

I was trying to take care of my bladder leakage issue when he started pounding on the door. I grabbed the broom I kept in the bathroom and began striking the wall with it. It hit the wall so hard that the handle flew off. I was in such a violent moment of rage. I used the exposed metal to scrape and cut at my wrists in an attempt to hurt myself. I was so out of control! I was in a full-blown state of rage.

My husband was at the door threatening to call the police if I didn't come out of the bathroom. I could hear my husband telling my son to call the police. When the police answered, he got scared and hung up the phone. Moments later, I heard my husband talking to dispatch explaining that I was okay just upset. Regardless they were sending an officer out. My husband said, "You better come out. The police are going to come now because Ezekiel hung up on them."

I knew what the process was in situations like this. The fear of being sent for a psychological evaluation and possibly being hospitalized snapped me out of my rage. I had scraped my wrists. I quickly wrapped the one that was bleeding more, grabbed my phone, my car keys, a bottle of water, and ran out the back door. My husband said, "Wait, you have to talk to the police when they get here." But that didn't stop me. I opened the back gate and walked to the park down the road.

I sat at the picnic table and tried to calm myself. I took deep breaths and hoped I would not cry because I didn't want to draw any attention to myself. Within five minutes, I noticed a police car driving in front of the park. I sat drinking my water. I wondered, *Is the officer going to turn the car around?* He did. I panicked but remained seated and looked at my phone as if I was surfing the web. The police officer kept driving and never came back. After I finished my water, I returned home to find out the officer visited my house to speak with my son and my husband. My husband explained that we argued, but I was fine and had gone for a walk. Thankfully, this incident did not escalate any further.

I knew I needed to do something more to overcome the aggression I was facing. I did some tapping that evening and yes, my husband's comment and the anger I felt because of the financial burden, were evident triggers. But I discovered, the trigger that pushed me to a state of rage was the bladder leakage. I realized that I felt hopeless because I thought, *How can I help myself if I can't even control my body?*

Another thing I want to point out is how rage has been a common theme in my life. As a child, I never felt safe because I never knew what was going to set it off. I thought, *If I could just be the perfect child and please everyone, they would be happy and not rage.* After a while, it affected me. I became grouchy. I remember my dad calling me Oscar the Grouch. I think about it now, and I believe I used this as a defense mechanism to control my reaction to the rage. I know it sounds crazy. But I thought, *Why try to be happy? It doesn't help anyway.*

I thought about my childhood that day. I realized the rage was the programming Nick Ortner talked about that I needed to change. Instantly, I knew tapping was working for me! It made me feel calm and safe. But I had so much against me because I resorted to rage. Also, my old programs directed me to use Western Medicine because that is all I knew.

On Halloween that year, I couldn't take it anymore. I explained to my doctor, "I'm becoming aggressive; I can't even stand myself." He responded, "I wouldn't have known you are feeling this way because you look calm." I requested some medication to help ease my chronic stress and aggression. I was asked to complete anxiety and depression questionnaires. I showed signs of moderate anxiety and mild depression according to the results. I wondered, *Is the Pregabalin causing my aggression?* I discussed the possibility of stopping the Pregabalin and tying Naltrexone. I read it helped with chronic pain especially bladder pain. My doctor prescribed Sertraline for my anxiety and depression. He told me it would take time to have an effect on me. I thought, *How much longer can I hold on?*

Here is an excerpt from my symptom log:

10/31/14-

9:00am—appt w/Dr. McRae. Shared clinical note/ recommendations of nasal surgery as per ENT doctor, AZ Active Chiro—Dr. Porterfield. Focus—Neck L side, *trapezius* (traps)/right (R) pectoralis(pec)/neck/cervical spine—no headaches past 7 days, 2/7 days pre-headache symptoms bilateral (B) /forehead, massage (deep tissue)/stretches w/Julie Wilson. Focus—upper body, cervical spine, neck, B pecs, Kempton & Nelson PT—Physical Therapy (PT) program focus on cervical spine/neck, R pec & rib # 4 & 5—spasms—(R Pec - 3/ 7 days—erector spinae 1/7 days), B latissimus dorsi (lats)/traps/rhomboids 0/7days), SWGI—Dr. Kaiser recommended lab work to retest liver enzymes, endoscopy 11/3/14 to rule out (r/o) peptic ulcer, pancreas, stomach, upper Gastro Enterology (GI) large intestine diagnosis (Dx) (took note of allergy test results 2/5/14, constipation, ureter inflammation CT 8/5/14) & con't *pantoprazole* & sucralfate. Discussed mood—aggression—inquired discharge (D/C) Pregabalin, trial LD Naltrexone? Completed anxiety & depression questionnaires (scored moderate (mod) anxiety, mild depression-trial prescription (Rx) Sertraline 50 mg). Reported no R side abdominal (ABD) pain, dizziness, or nausea last 7 days. Gastroesophageal reflux disease GERD daily even w/Rx meds, added magnesium different brand without (w/o) rice flour & trialed pea protein—noted increased mod burning sensation 10/29/14, con't magnesium 10/30/14 very slight burning sensation. F/U with w/ AZ Asthma/ Allergy—Nicole Englert, PA, to request (req) test for food items noted in symptom log, referral to San Tan Allergy & Asthma/Dr. Jain RE: req for nasal/sinus swab/culture due to con't concern for nasal/sinus swab to r/o fungus/virus. Dr. McRae—administered trigger point injections (lidocaine hydrochloride) to B Traps/Lats/erectors & lidocaine hydrochloride/steroid R pec & F/U 11/06/14 1pm. Weight (Wt): 102.2 Blood Pressure (BP): 101/66

I figured, *Maybe I could use tapping to bridge that gap from old to new.* So, I kept tapping! :)

But every day, I had a constant reminder of my actions. I saw the dents in the walls of my bathroom. I felt tormented, guilty, ashamed, and sad. I completed another self-development course that year. The topic was to make your house feel like a sanctuary. The activity was to remove any physical items that cause you distress. I removed several things but did nothing to repair the bathroom walls.

Several times since that day, I have thought about making those repairs so I can finally release this troubling event from my past. To thoroughly enjoy the calm and safety that I am blessed to experience every time I tap. I am happy to report I can move forward with my life. I restored my bathroom walls along with my body, mind, soul, and spirit in 2017!

Healing Insight 4: Toxic relationships have to go!

All Thought Leaders

I always knew and agreed with this basic concept. However, I didn't think it applied to family members. I thought it was exclusively for bad romantic relationships, friendships, business relationships, but not family. I questioned, *How can you end a relationship with your family even if it is toxic?* I learned family was important and came first. I struggled with this concept because of the relationship I had with my mother. I had been trying to maintain a civil relationship with her until May of 2012. Even though I haven't spoken to her since that date, I have had difficulty processing all the guilt, shame, resentment, anger, disappointment, hurt, sadness, sorrow, and grief. As I continued my journey with self development courses, this concept—toxic relationships must go—was discussed by every thought leader.

Even though I had essentially cut ties with my mother since 2012, I still felt bound to the negative emotion. The fact that we lived in different states made it somewhat easier, but my heart continued to ache. Because I had difficulty with forgiveness, it made the process of healing especially challenging. Even after reading *The Power of Your Subconscious Mind* by Joseph Murphy and applying the process of forgiveness to the relationship with my mother, these emotions haunted me and would surface time and time again!

In one self-development course, the activity was to write a thank-you list about a family member. For example, Thank you for_____. It was not expected that you would send this list to the other person. They would never have to know. It was a way of you placing your energy on the positive instead of the negative aspects of the relationship. I cried as I wrote the thank-you list. I had to wipe my tears off the paper before I placed it in a folder. My thank-you list was for my mother.

A year after I wrote the thank-you list, I found it when I was looking for some papers. I reread the list as tears streamed down my face. For a whole week, I contemplated whether I should send the list to my mother or not. Finally, I built up the courage, wrote with love, signed my name to it, and sent it off. Initially, I felt good about my actions. But then I realized the can of worms I opened up.

My mother attempted to reach me by having other family members convince me to call her. I had sent my brother a birthday card in October. I had forgotten to leave my address off the envelope. So, when my mother received this list in November the week before Thanksgiving, she had access to my address when my brother took his card home. She had him send me a belated birthday card to see if the address was correct. Then she sent a letter in response to my thank-you list. The message had a mixture of positive and negative comments. Several pictures accompanied it. Mostly, of my children, myself, my husband, and a few with her or my father along with my family. One of the pictures was cut in half. I suppose in the attempt to cut it up, but she just didn't finish the job.

All the work I had done seemed pointless. I felt like kicking myself for sending the thank-you list. I disconnected even more with my mother's side of the family. I didn't want her to hound them or try to make me contact her. I continued to struggle with these emotions up until summer 2017. In another self-development course, by Iyanla Vanzant, an activity was titled, "What's the Matter with You?" The point of this activity was to quiet my critical voice and any limiting beliefs still holding me back.

Here are my answers to that activity.

Who Are You?
I am me
I am happy
I am confident
I am strong
I am beautiful
I am courageous
I am smart
I am loving
I am kind

What's the matter with you?
I am too hard on myself, not worthy of my mother's love so how can I love myself. How does this threaten you? It makes me feel guilty

Index card-front side.

Breakfast incident
"Don't spend $ all in one place"
Stress about $ reaching 30 sale day!
They got right programs I didn't
It's too late!?
I don't deserve financial freedom
$ incident @ Sonic felt stupid
I can do more, I am better
I'm not sure body, mind will maintain
NO, security stopping me
Learned love fake, hurtful, mean
I not worthy of love like dad
You just settle for the crap you have get
My false belief around $ worthy/mom
addicted to misery

Relationships/Finances

Index card-back side.

As you can see I still had so much guilt, shame, resentment, hatred, hurt, sadness, sorrow, and grief. One morning, I was feeling rushed and frustrated because my hair wasn't doing what I wanted it to do. I felt that same feeling of not being able to stand myself the way I felt when I was so aggressive in October 2014. I became enraged! I realized I was yanking on my hair, so I started tapping forcefully on the wrist point as I stood in front of the mirror. I cried, screamed, and let out every true statement about how I was feeling!

Every negative comment I ever heard from my critical voice came out that day. Positive statements were hard to find. When I did express something that was somewhat positive, it was wrapped with sarcasm. When I finished tapping, my wrists hurt, bruised from tapping so hard. But strangely since that day forward, I felt an overall sense of well-being. I felt cleansed. I felt free. I felt safe and I felt calm. I don't know if I will experience those emotions related to the relationship I've had with my mother ever again. But if I do, I know what to do. I will tap to find the hope, the healing, and the peace.

Healing Insight 5: Journaling creates action!

Awaken the Giant Within, Tony Robbins

Boy, Tony Robbins said a mouthful when he said, "Take massive action!" He also emphasizes, "You get what you focus on in life," in his book, *Awaken the Giant Within.* This book offers journaling opportunities which prove to be valuable to the process of healing. I realized journaling creates action as I accepted his invitation to journal. Maybe it was his stern, commanding voice on the audiobook that convinced me. Or perhaps it was the inspiration that flowed from his positive energy. Whatever motivated me, I did take massive action!

I attempted to journal when I was in my twenties. I was encouraged by my sister-in-law to keep a daily journal to list what I was thankful for at the end of each day. It was something that Oprah Winfrey recommended on her talk show. I tried this, but I wasn't feeling it. It seemed so repetitious and even tedious so unfortunately, I stopped doing it after about a week. As I think back, I wonder, *Why I didn't feel the need to continue journaling*? I have always been one to take notes because I am a visual learner and I can see the written pages in my memory when I need to recall information. But somehow, the daily task of journaling didn't keep my interest.

I think journaling works for me now because I don't realize what I am doing. I see it as merely completing an activity on a page. Writing a quote that touched my heart. Or listing tips or steps I want to remember from self-development courses I have participated in during this process. I now have two binders, three spiral notebooks, several note cards, a journal (the war room journal), as well as a gratitude jar.

There is only one spiral I tore up and threw away during this healing process. It was the very first journal experience I had while I was on the *10-Day Detox Diet.* I kept the spiral for over a year. I even reread it once I finished. It was an eye-opener; it was inspirational. It was proof of how far I had come and how much further I needed to go.

I asked my husband to read it because it was just too complicated for me to express so much of what I felt during that time. He started reading it, but I don't think he ever finished because it was quite lengthy. It included the *10-Day Detox Diet* plus the six-week extended plan journal notes. I finally shredded it one day while I was cleaning up around the house. I was a bit hurt my husband never finished reading it. I think that's what prompted me to shred it. I only wish I had saved it, so I could share it with you.

As I look back on this journey, I'm so grateful I am a woman of my word. When I say I'm going to do something, I have great follow-through. Also, I'm incredibly open-minded. I'm not afraid to try new techniques. My experience working with children with autism spectrum disorder proved to me no matter how ridiculous the method seemed if you applied it, if you used it, it worked. So please do not disregard the activities in personal-development books as a way to take up space on a page.

A quote from Dr. Joe Dispenza: "Think of it this way: The input remains the same, so the output has to remain the same. How then can you ever create anything new?"

I have completed every activity in these miraculous books I have read. I didn't realize that the process of journaling is so beneficial. It allows you to make a neurological connection to the motor action. The physical part of writing, which is considered meditative journaling, has many benefits. It is known to make learning easier, improve memory, help you be in the present moment, and make your goals a reality. I have learned all successful people write their goals because they can see and feel the words come to life. Also, they can refer to their journal for inspiration, for encouragement, and for proof that they have endured, succeeded, and mastered these goals.

Remember, you have two minds: the conscious and the subconscious mind. The conscious mind creates the plan, and the subconscious mind carries it out. When you journal, your conscious mind creates the thoughts which become feelings. Then your subconscious mind takes those feelings and carries them out, turning them into action. When you know this bit of knowledge, you can use it along with the benefits of journaling to create the life you deserve.

Allow your conscious mind to create the plan for a goal. See how your subconscious mind carries out that goal and turns it into a reality. When your body, mind, soul, and spirit are tuned in to your thoughts, feelings, and actions, your life will change! Once this happens, remember how you felt when you rehearsed making your goal a reality. These feelings are the connection between thoughts and actions which cause changes to take place. Starting in your body, then in your life, and the world around you.

No, I'm not saying to journal every day. Start with once a week. If that works for you, stick to it. If you feel the need to journal two or three times a week, then feel free to do that. Make it work for you. Don't just write why you are grateful. Journal what your critical voice is telling you. Be honest with how you're feeling. Create a goal to work on and read it every day or every time you journal. This routine along with a positive thought will set your goal in motion. Now start feeling how it would feel if your goal would become a reality.

The Activities and/or Daily Challenges throughout the book are
compliments of the Healing Insights 70-Day Course.

Activity:

Instructions:

"On Your Mark, Get Set, Journal!"

Let's start journaling right now. Enjoy this activity. You are creating a goal and a life you desire. Make it real!

- Write down a goal you would like to work on.

- Now take it a step further.

- Include details that include the five senses.

- What are you wearing?

- What do you see?

- What do you smell?

- What do you hear?

- What do you feel with your sense of touch?

- Now go even further!

- How do you feel (emotion)?

- How will you behave?

- What will you experience?

- What state of mind will you be in?

Journal Tips:

- Start With 1x Per Week.

- Stick to It.

- Be Honest!

Journal Tips Checklist

	Be Sure to Include the Following
	Express Feelings (Emotions)
	Express Gratitude
	Release Critical Voice
	Release False Beliefs
	Create a Goal
	Read Goal Every Day!

Healing Insight 6: Try different things.

Brooke Love, PT, AZ Urogynecology

This healing insight is so basic it almost sounds like common sense. However, when your body is in a state of constant stress, you can't access your common sense. Brain fog is a symptom of fibromyalgia which clouds even the most basic decisions you must make. When I was receiving pelvic floor therapy, I was reminded I could try different things. With IBS and a spastic pelvic floor, I had severe constipation. I discussed this with my therapist. I followed my primary doctor's suggestions, but I had little success.

One day my therapist inquired about my status. I mentioned to her things were about the same. I was still backed up. That's when she said, "You can try different things, remember not everyone responds to treatment the same way." She gave me the name of a tea I could try. Also, she suggested I try different constipation regimens. She said, "It's worth the effort because you might just find something that works for you and if you don't try different things then you may never find a solution."

During that timeframe, an activity I was doing for a self-development course asked, "If you were given six months to live, what would you do in your life every single day to feel alive?" My answer was yoga, meditation, and eating healthy. The next question was, "Why do you have to wait until you're dying to make improvements in your life?" Right? This activity couldn't have come at a better time since the door had already been opened for me to try different things!

As simple as this seems, I was so stuck in the stress response cycle that I couldn't even think straight. But I did start trying new things. The tea didn't work. The other constipation regimen did give me some relief. But it was the diet changes that seemed to give me the most relief. I was both happy and intrigued by this simple insight 'you can try new things,' because it gave me permission to explore other techniques, treatments, and remedies. At the time, I thought about the scientific process I was taught in school. The concept is this. You basically ask a question, make an educated guess (hypothesis), and then conduct an experiment to see if you're right; so simple, right?

I kept trying new things. I searched YouTube for five-minute yoga videos. Yes, that is correct, five-minute yoga videos because I was severely fatigued, my endurance was low, and my pain was extreme. I knew I had to start small. Some keywords I used included: for beginners, easy, restorative, and low flexibility.

I explored new techniques, treatments, and remedies. It made me feel empowered! It gave me some control of my life. It gave me the responsibility for my own care. Now I was the scientist conducting the experiments. If something didn't work, I just said, "Oh well, it was worth a try." If it did work and I did find some relief, I took note. I paid attention so I could get more relief. I added what worked to my daily life so I could turn it into a healthy habit.

I will share with you a list of some of the treatments, techniques, and remedies. I have experimented with many. Some of them may seem silly and extreme. But I have gotten so much relief from these techniques, I have made them part of my healthy lifestyle. I will highlight some of my favorites and tell you why they're my favorite and how exactly they helped me to heal my mind, body, soul, and spirit!

Forty days of Kundalini Yoga for compassion. Yes, I did all forty days! I truly enjoyed Kundalini Yoga (or active yoga) because it includes movement along with mantras. Mantras are words or phrases that have sacred meaning and are repeated several times. My top two mantras are Teyata Om and Adi Shakti. Teyata means going beyond (Samsara and Nirvana). Om means jewel holder, wish fulfilling one, auspicious one. It is a mantra to release negative energy and promote health. Adi Shakti, Namo Namo means I bow to primal power. This mantra is used to tap into the creative power of manifestation in the universe. I also tried energy cleansing, Qi Gong, and chakra meditations.

Stuck in a chronic stress response cycle, I needed to cleanse my entire energy system from negative thoughts and self-limiting beliefs. These techniques, treatments, and remedies are part of my daily lifestyle now. I also signed up for email newsletters from MyFitnessPal. I had downloaded their APP on my phone when I started the *10-Day Detox Diet* in 2014. This APP was perfect because it sent me information and videos including yoga, exercise, health tips, and recipes.

I needed this type of support. Remember, signing up for email newsletters has many advantages. I will provide a full list of those individuals I follow and receive newsletters from in the resource section of this book. I hope you will take responsibility for your health, self-care, and eating habits to improve your lifestyle. Believe it or not, you are worth it!

Healing Insight 7: What BS story are you telling yourself?

Awaken the Giant Within, Tony Robbins

Again, I hear Tony Robbins' words in my ears: "What BS story are you telling yourself?" He sure knows how to get his point across. This statement was precisely phrased to get a response. I was intrigued by what he was going to talk about. He went on to explain we all have a BS story, holding us back. We tell ourselves and others this BS story so often, we begin to believe it.

That is why your thoughts matter. You say to yourself, "I would start that exercise, but I can't because I work. I need to pick up the kids from school. I need go to the grocery store, and I need to cook dinner.

So, I don't have any spare time." As a result, you don't start your exercise program. You are using excuses, even if they are true, according to Tony Robbins' statement. This statement almost seems insulting, right? But his purpose is to grab your attention and make you think. His comment made me ask myself, *What have I been telling myself and others? How have I been limiting myself? How have I been keeping myself from having a wonderful life? What statements am I hiding behind?*

You also must remember what you tell yourself and other people sets the Law of Attraction into motion. Let me give you an example: You think the thought, *I don't have any time.* Then you feel rushed, which makes you believe there really is a lack of time. The result, you don't have any time! This cycle of negative thoughts equals negative feelings that lead to negative actions which become a reality.

I know you genuinely have a lot to do, and you feel pressed for time. It does seem hard to find time for yourself. I struggled with this because I always put myself last. I didn't listen to the aches and pains in my body. I didn't realize my critical voice needed to be quieted. I didn't want to face the fact I needed to learn the process of forgiveness. I pushed through the pain. I didn't even know at the time that I didn't have any coping skills to process all the emotions stuck in my body causing me physical, emotional, and spiritual pain. I hope I stress how important self-care is in this process of healing. I know how hard it is even to think straight when you're not feeling well, and your body is screaming with pain. Not to mention always being tired, stressed out, frustrated, and confused.

"Don't think can't, think how… turn BUTS into AND."

~Phil Lector~

When I heard this quote from Phil Lector, Vice President of Tecademics, at the TEC Talks 2017 Conference I applied it to my BS story to change BUT to AND. It's simple! Turn *but* into *and* so you can create a positive Law of Attraction cycle to improve your life.

Say this: "I've been trying to start that exercise, and I'm going to figure out how I can fit it into my schedule." Remember everyone has the same twenty-four hours. What amazing things are you going to do with yours? It's encouraging when you finally realize how much power you really have. You can create a pain-free life and love every minute of it!

One other thing you must remember is anytime you say, "I can't," your brain automatically shuts down. Then you can't think of any solutions. On the flipside, if you say, "How can I make time?" your brain automatically sees the possibilities. So, it's like this, you say, "How can I find the time to do my exercise program?" You automatically feel the hope. You can find a solution, and you make time! Do you see how the BS story you've been telling yourself and others can be changed?

Let me assure you the Law of Attraction is as real as the Law of Gravity! We use it every day, we are just not aware of what it is. We can use it to create anything we desire. The simple thought of wanting coffee in the morning makes you feel invigorated, right, because you know how it will taste. You sense how it will feel energizing and how warm it will make your body. The flavor is so good, so you get up out of bed, and you start that coffee pot. This series of events is the Law of Attraction in action. You had a positive thought and felt a positive feeling, so you made it happen. In the beginning, it was an intentional process, right? Yes, you really had to think about it. Then after several repetitions, that daily cup of coffee became a daily habit.

Now use the Law of Attraction cycle to your advantage! This is exactly how you can create a healthy habit. Think a positive thought, send out the positive energy, and feel the emotions as if it were already a reality. This process will create positive action because your conscious mind created the plan and the subconscious mind must carry it out. Notice how positive changes will take place in your body—and in your life. Focus on action. You can't expect change without changing your BS story! It just won't happen.

Healing Insight 8: You have to see the dirt before you can clean it up.

Author Louise Hay couldn't have said it any better: "You have to see the dirt before you can clean it up." I think this is one of the hardest things to be able to do. It's so easy for us to see faults in others. To see what others need to improve in their lives. To understand why other people's lives are not going in the right direction. To see others stuck in patterns of bad behaviors and habits. Seeing the dirt may be possibly the hardest step in the healing process, but if we ever expect to start making changes, we must see the dirt.

It was not easy for me to see and especially difficult for me to accept that my life was a mess. I believe we all know what we need to work on deep down. It's that level of acceptance that gets in the way of us cleaning up our mess. Why do you think it is so hard for us to see the dirt? Again, it is common sense. A core concept you must comprehend and accept before you can move forward.

Let's retake a closer look at how our brain and body function. Did you know that 95% of the day the subconscious mind takes over and operates your brain and body? This statistic was based on the books *Biology of Belief* by Dr. Bruce Lipton and *You Are the Placebo by* Dr. Joe Dispenza. That means you're only aware 5% of the day when your conscious mind is active and present. That means 95% of the time your subconscious mind is running your programs and habits. This process is efficient, saves energy, and has allowed you to survive.

The thing is, false beliefs, ridicule, and programs that aren't even yours undermine your routine and habits. Programs that you picked up along the way throughout your life. This process would be great if you had habits that were nurturing, loving, and positive. But for the most part, the habits that are being run by your subconscious mind 95% of the day are bad habits. These habits keep you stuck in the past, keep you anchored to addiction, and prevent you from achieving a full life.

People are unable to see the dirt because of this. For example, when people are acting like their parents did, they can't see their behavior. When they're in the moment of acting like their parent and running that old program, they are not aware. They are not using their conscious mind, and their subconscious mind is running the show. So, they are unable to remain aware even if they do notice the dirt when they are conscious. That is what happens the other 95% of the day when their subconscious returns to old beliefs, old programs, and bad habits!

I know this sounds grim when you first realize it. Maybe that's why only 1% of people succeed with self-development (as noted in Tai Lopez's *67 Steps*). Yes, an excellent course is designed and structured to help them succeed. So why don't they? They don't triumph because they never learned how the mind and the body function. But there is hope! The mind can be changed. Habits can be changed. If you know how your body and brain work, you can use this insight to your advantage, and create and live a full life that you deserve.

Another critical factor that I must discuss is the fact that 80% of your thoughts are negative every day. Also 98% of the time you are having the same exact thoughts that you had the day before. Please read that last sentence again. (More stats noted in Dr. Bruce Lipton and Dr. Joe Dispenza's books.) Let me clarify a bit more, with an example from my life. I woke up and the first thought was, *Oh, f*** my life sucks, I feel like a 90-year-old woman, my life is a joke, I want to be dead.* At least I prayed and was grateful for my family. So now let's apply the stats to show you the process of getting stuck in old programs and bad habits every day.

As you can see 80% of my thoughts were negative, therefore, 98% of the time, I had the same exact negative thought every day. I was astonished when I heard this! I was shaken. I thought, *Wow, I really, don't have a chance if I continue having the same thoughts, the same feelings, and doing the same thing every day of my life.* I hope this will shake you up, grab your attention, and make you listen! I want to help you understand, dig deep, find your inner strength, and see the hope. Plan to change your thoughts. Change how you feel and change your life today!

A bit more insight to motivate you: the brain doesn't know whether a habit is good or bad. I learned this nugget of information from a book to develop positive programs and good habits into your life titled *The Power of Habit* by Charles Duhigg. You must remember your subconscious mind is going to run your programs and habits 95% of the day. Also, remember 98% of the time you will be thinking the same thoughts as you did the day before. So, they might as well be positive programs and good habits, right? Once you get these positive programs and good habits in place, the odds are for you and not against you.

Another tidbit of information: you must see the triggers in order to change a habitual pattern. Understanding how the brain and body function is going to help you figure out why it's happening.

Healing Insight 9: Your environment affects you.

All Thought Leaders

This healing insight takes me back to my college studies. I learned this concept as nature versus nurture. I had the basic idea. But I would figure out to what extent the environment could affect you. This insight perfectly reinforces the fact that lifestyle causes illness 95% of the time. Remember, genetics only account for medical conditions 5% of the time.

In 2012, when I first stopped working due to my multiple medical conditions, my husband and I were both at home. He had been working from home and hated it. He was frustrated with his situation just as much as I was with mine. Every day we got up angry. We were bitter. We were hateful, and we were rude. I asked him, "Damn, can you feel the oppression, the suppression, and the depression in this house?"

We wouldn't even say good morning or acknowledge the other existed. I complained and griped about my body and how awful it felt. I grabbed my medications, took them after I ate, and I was out for several hours. After the drowsiness wore off, I woke up, griped a bit more, ate, took my prescriptions, and got knocked out again. For the brief time I was awake and not drugged up sleeping on my couch, my husband and I argued and were rude with one another.

Even though I could feel the suppression, oppression, and depression in my home, I had no idea how deeply it was affecting me. I did not realize to what level it had consumed my thoughts, feelings, and life. It had changed my mind, body, soul, and crushed my spirit. Sadly, this pattern continued for the next two years. It wasn't until 2014 when I started my journey of self-development that I realized I had to change my environment. One self-development activity suggested removing physical items from the environment that might be causing you distress.

This activity was a good start. Little did I know that my environment was more than just the physical realm. I was also affected by mental torture caused by self-inflicted negative thoughts. This emotional breakdown of not being able to release two decades of grief, sadness, sorrow, anger, hatred, disgust, resentment, guilt, and shame was a huge factor. Not to mention, the environmental effects on my body. Like all the poison I ate that I considered food. Also, the lack of consistent physical activity and exercise. The stress that had built up around my ever-increasing financial burden played a part, too. I was a walking time bomb ready to explode at any moment! I remember marching into my living room and declaring to my husband, "I hate my life, and I hate who I have become. I don't know how I'm going to do it, but something has to change."

Again, I would like to emphasize how the environment affects you. I continue to unravel the layers and the depths at which the environment affects you. It wasn't until late summer of 2017 when I finished a book called *The Book of Secrets* by Bhagwan Shree Rajneesh. I came to understand how compelling both positive and negative environments can be. As I read the paragraph that explained how we affect one another with our energy system it cemented this healing insight to be true.

The author explained how a person that is depressed could walk into the room and change the mood of everyone, despite their best attempt to appear happy and okay. On the flip side of that, he also explained how a genuinely enlightened person could also affect other people in the environment, and the effect is much more significant because the positive energy is stronger, balanced, and healthy. He went on to describe how positive energy can affect and be felt by other individuals up to 24 miles away. That's mind-blowing! It's hard to grasp. How can this be?

"It is really not possible to discover your purpose if you are depleted and not full."

~Oprah Winfrey~

This effect must be what Oprah Winfrey describes as being full of yourself. She describes it as, "I'm so full that my cup runneth over." She went on to say, "I believe you will never have enough to give unless you keep your own self full. That means honoring yourself. Your real job on earth beyond the minutes, hours, and days is to keep your cup full." We are spiritual beings with energy systems. When our energy systems are balanced, and the chakra centers are clear, that positive energy can go out into the environment and be felt deeply by others.

It makes sense: a person that is enlightened has nurtured the body, the mind, the soul, and the spirit in every sense of the environment. That person has created a space to heal by priming the parasympathetic nervous system. That person has achieved what I learned in college as homeostasis, a state of balance and well-being. We can all attain this balance and prosperity; it is not something that has to evade us. It is not so far away that we cannot reach it. We have the ability inside of us to create a space to heal to have health, wealth, love, and happiness.

We must start by realizing what type of energy is in our environment and how it is affecting us. How are we affecting others in return? We must recognize that we are able to influence others around us in such a positive way that they can feel it even if they are 24 miles away! That's amazing! That day my only thought was, *Wow I want to be the person that can affect people 24 miles away from me*!

Healing Insight 10: Tapping meditation is one of the four ways to change your programs.

The Tapping Solution Documentary Film, Dr. Bruce Lipton

I used to think I was just stumbling upon these great resources by chance or by some stroke of luck. But now as I have continued to choose to be an abundant thinker, I realize it is true that you see things more clearly when your energy is focused on something. Because I was focused on 'Tapping,' I was able to gain this insight from reading Dr. Bruce Lipton's book, *Biology of Belief*. I had already been introduced to Dr. Lipton by Nick Ortner because he is one of the doctors that endorsed EFT Tapping in *The Tapping Solution* Documentary Film.

It wasn't until my oldest son and I were having a conversation about some of the great thought leaders that each of us had been following, when we realized that we were both so intrigued by Dr. Bruce Lipton, my son suggested that I read Dr. Lipton's book. I did because I was already so fascinated by what he had to say about 'Tapping.' Dr. Lipton explained, "EFT engages the process of super learning." He described super learning as, "The process of pushing the record button on the subconscious mind." So, what are the four ways to change your programs?

According to Dr. Lipton, "The four ways are hypnosis, repetition, energy psychology (which EFT 'Tapping' is considered) and high-impact events such as traumatizing life-changing events that make us realize we need or want to change like a near-death experience or having a terminal illness." This helped me to understand how 'Tapping' could be used for anything and everything in my life!

I also thought what a wonderful gift 'Tapping' is, because it gave me a feeling of safety, calm. Plus, it's free! I was truly feeling empowered. I had discovered the most amazing healing technique ever! Not only did I now have a coping skill to process and release my emotions, I also had a tool to change my old programs. I had a way to feel calm and safe, so I could create a space to heal my mind, my body, my soul, and my spirit!

Now I was starting to understand how the process of 'Tapping' worked. I was super excited that I was equipped with what I needed to change everything I hated about my life and who I had become. I was ready to release thoughts, emotions, and events in my past. I shared this information with my sons and my husband. I felt like a kid again because I felt like I had a second chance. I felt like I was training for my comeback. I was ready for the responsibility that I had for my own life for my health, wealth, love, and happiness. I had lost so much. I had lost hope. I had lost self-respect. I had lost my will to live. I had lost connections with my family. I had lost my ability to heal.

The thought of winning all of this back and creating a life that I loved and that I deserved—that astonished me! I hadn't heard any of this. I had never learned this in any of the years I had been educated (not at any level). Yes, I had been taught to have faith. I had been taught that love could carry you through anything. I had been taught that if you just persevere, you can achieve. But I had not been taught how the mind works. I had not been taught how the body works. I had not been taught how to access this super learning process. I had not been taught to participate in the creation of my own life.

I was amazed at how much control I had of actually changing my own life! I started 'Tapping' about everything. I couldn't get enough. I also quickly learned that what I thought was my issue was just the tip of the iceberg. I had to dive deep into those emotions. I had to relive those events. I had to be willing to let emotions pour out. When I did, the slate was cleared and I felt joy! I felt calm! I felt hope, healing, and peace!

I also want to share how this journey of mine continues to be a process. It wasn't until October of 2017 when I was reading Dr. Joe Dispenza's book *Evolve Your Brain* that I had a deeper level of awareness of how and why 'Tapping' works. Dr. Dispenza explained, "The amygdala (the stress center of the brain) stores aggression, joy, sadness, and fear." This helped me to understand how detrimental the stress response cycle really is.

This new understanding helped me realize that I had been stuck in the stress response cycle for too long. I could see how I was storing aggression, sadness, and fear in my amygdala. This new information enlightened me. This is why I feel the pure joy and elation when I 'Tap'. I hope this encourages you to realize what has taken me so long. Your body is equipped with everything you need to heal! You just need to understand how your mind and your body work so that you can change those programs, those thoughts, those emotions, and those events that are holding you back from taking back your health, taking control of your life, and finding relief!

Healing Insight 11: So what do you think you did wrong?

Dr. Porterfield, AZ Active Chiropractic

I was asked this question by my sports medicine chiropractor. This is the same chiropractor to whom I give credit for me being able to attend my youngest son's high school graduation. I had a week-long migraine which caused me to seek medical attention at the ER and Urgent Care in May 2014. I was so weak and fatigued after losing another five pounds. Dr. Porterfield helped relieve the pain in my neck and my head so that I could feel better and get rid of my migraine. I also got my appetite back.

This healing insight prompted me to take a deep look at what I did wrong, what wasn't working for me, and why I needed to see what wasn't working. If I expected my life to get better, I could not continue to think the same, feel the same, and do the same things. I'm a bit embarrassed by the answer that I gave my chiropractor when he asked me, "So what do you think you did wrong?" It was around the time when my liver enzymes were elevated, my digestive system was a mess, and I was allergic to 42 different foods. My response to him was, "I ate too much quinoa." I know, right, what does that have to do with all of those issues? Absolutely—nothing!

I wasn't even capable of being aware, being able to accept and face the fact that I was clueless about nutrition. I'm sure he wanted to laugh, but he didn't. I hadn't been eating quinoa forever. Quinoa was the new food in my diet to replace wheat. Yes, maybe I was eating it more than I should have because it's a starch. But it was not what led to all of these issues in any way, shape, or form. As I think back on this healing insight, I can see how stuck I was. I couldn't even go beyond what I was experiencing. I wasn't willing to look in the mirror and take responsibility. I couldn't see the dirt.

I wasn't taught proper nutrition like many of us. We were all watching the same commercials and following the same guidelines, which I have come to find out are very misleading and influenced for the sole purpose of profit. At the time, I just felt stupid. I felt embarrassed. I felt angry because I didn't know the first thing about a healthy meal. My childhood was littered with sweets, wheat, and sodas.

Here is a sample of what I ate daily.

Breakfast:

As a child, my breakfast consisted of red rope licorice, Lucky Charms, Fruity Pebbles, Raisin Bran, Frosted Flakes, Frosted Mini Wheats, Grandma's brand or Little Debbie cookies.

As a teen, my breakfast consisted of pizza pockets, Cinnamon Bears, Pepsi, Nibs (red licorice).

As an adult, my breakfast consisted of large cinnamon rolls with icing, Pop Tarts, granola bars, hot tea with 2-3 teaspoons sugar, flavored instant oatmeal, and wheat toast.

Lunch:

As a child, my lunch was a school lunch during the week. On the weekend it was a TV dinner. Or a full-meal deal from Dairy Queen which included hot dogs, hamburgers, French fries, Pepsi, and an ice cream.

As a teen, my lunch was pizza, grilled cheese, canned soup, a deli meat sandwich with cheese, lettuce, pickles, a SPAM sandwich (w/tortilla), an occasional salad with Catalina dressing, cheese, and croutons, Pepsi, and hot tamales or licorice.

As an adult my lunch was ramen noodles, peanut butter and jelly sandwiches, chips, steak sandwiches from Sonic or extra-long Coney with tater tots, Pepsi, an occasional side salad, and baked potato with sour cream, chives, and cheese from Wendy's, and Starburst or some other type of chewy candy.

Dinner:

As a child, my dinner was mostly meat and potato or tortilla-based meals, canned veggies (usually corn, carrots, or peas) a Sonic kid's meal, 7 Up or Cherry 7 Up.

As a teen my dinner was TV dinners, fast-food meals, restaurant meals; since my mom was working outside the home now common meals were hot open-faced turkey, beef, or steak with mashed potatoes, loads of gravy, rolls, canned veggies, a side salad with salad dressing, cheese, croutons, iced tea with diet sweetener, and Kool-Aid with loads of sugar.

As an adult my dinner was chili fries, Mexican burgers (burger/cheese on tortilla, French fries with red chili to dip fries in), steak sandwiches from Sonic with tater tots, cherry limeade or a slush, roast beef sandwiches from Arby's, French fries, Pepsi, iced tea with diet sweetener, and Kool-Aid with loads of sugar.

Snacks:

As a child, my snacks were sweet rice with sugar and cinnamon, cinnamon bears, licorice, chips, cookies, ice cream, hard candy, bubble gum, slushies, Pepsi, root-beer floats, homemade French fries, canned pineapple, mandarin oranges, and fruit cocktail in heavy corn syrup.

As a teen, my snacks were nachos with cheese, hot fries, pork skin chips, Funyuns, Bugles, Hot Tamales, Jolly Rancher candy, homemade French fries, canned pineapple, mandarin oranges, and fruit cocktail in heavy corn syrup.

As an adult, my snacks were hot tamales, red licorice, jerky, Chex Mix, Gardetto's, various processed cheese and crackers, dry sweet cereal, cookies, hard candy, canned pineapple, mandarin oranges, and fruit cocktail in heavy corn syrup.

Throughout my life I used all the condiments you can imagine—mustard, BBQ sauce, salad dressing, ketchup, mayo, butter, and I always added more sugar and salt to anything I ate.

As a child, I made trips to my Aunt Lucy's neighborhood general/candy store daily.

As a teen and adult, I drank 6-8 sweetened drinks per day, mostly Pepsi.

Don't get me wrong. I did eat plenty of fruits. Green apples right off the neighbor's tree; strawberries from my grandmother's garden; plums off our own trees and watermelon, cantaloupe, and honeydew from my grandfather's, produce truck. My parents always had fresh apples, oranges, lemons, limes, bananas, grapes, nectarines, and peaches for us. They also had some veggies—cucumbers, avocados, and pumpkin from our garden. We also grew squash and tomatoes, but I disliked them at the time.

My parents were so excited to be doing better financially around the year 1981, especially after a rough time when my father injured his back in the coal mine and was fighting for disability benefits. Once his settlement came through we had a microwave and all that junk to go with it. Also, I think they felt as if we had gone without so much. It was a time to enjoy the good stuff. Little did I know, the so-called good stuff was robbing me of the very nutrients and vitamins I needed.

It is no wonder I had a list of diagnoses a whole page long.

Diagnosis List

Left Sciatica	2003 Re-diagnosed 10-2012
Allergies	(Seasonal Lifetime)
Asthma	2008
Allergies Food Potato	2008
Chronic Pain	5/2012
Interstitial Cystitis	9/2012
Allergies (medication Percocet)	4/2013
Severe Vitamin D Deficiency	1/2013
Chronic Fatigue	1/2013
Irritable Bowel Syndrome	5/2013
Headache/Migraines	5/2013
Hiatus Hernia	6/2013
Central Sensitivity Syndrome with Fibromyalgia	7/2013
TMJ disorder	11/2013
Allergies Food 29 items	2/2014
Trigeminal Neuralgia	3/19/14
Arthritis Bilateral TMJ	3/25/14
Pinched Nerve @ C5 C6 vertebrae	3/18/14
Anemia	4/25/14 resolved 7/21/14
Allergies Food Additional 16 items	12/2/2014
Spastic Pelvic Floor Syndrome (PFTN) Pelvic Floor Tension Myalgia	11/10/14
Anemia	11/11/14 resolved 6/16/15
Endometriosis	1/2/15

I thought my body had fought and healed from the multiple surgeries and medical procedures that I have had throughout my life. But it didn't.

Surgery List

1987	Episiotomy
1990	Tonsillectomy
1993	Tubal Ligation
2002	Exploratory Laparoscopy
2002	Vaginal Hysterectomy, Rectocele
2003	Left Salpingo Oophorectomy
2012	Cystocele, Rectocele, Transvaginal Intraperitoneal Enterocele Repair, Cystoscopy & Hydrodistension
2014	Left Breast Incisional Biopsy Benign
2015	Exploratory Laparoscopy (lysis of adhesions, removal of endometriosis, cyst right ovary), Cystoscopy, Hydrodistension (extended 30 minutes)
2016	Cystoscopy, Hydrodistension (extended 30 minutes)

Not to mention, the energy was drained from my body from all the stress, the emotions, and the events in my life that I did not know how to cope with. So, the question, "What do you think you did wrong?" was exactly what I needed at that time in my life.

I needed to evaluate what I was putting into my body. Not just food, but what thoughts I was putting into my mind. What feelings I was storing—in my heart and in my brain. What events were holding me back from healing. I can't stress enough how the process of healing must include your mind, body, soul, and spirit! I hope you will remember that.

Here is a sample of what I eat now.

Breakfast:

My breakfasts consist of quinoa, buckwheat, raw nut cereal with fruit, decaf coffee (with coconut milk, stevia, and pea protein powder,) sourdough or sprouted grain toast with raw cashew butter and fruit, or eggs with vegetables.

Lunch:

My lunch includes salads, vegetable soup, veggie sandwiches, raw or roasted vegetables, hummus and sprouted crackers

Dinner:

I regularly eat veggie-based meals that include legumes (beans), quinoa, salad, soup, salsa, and guacamole dip.

Snacks:

The snacks I keep on hand are fruit/nut bars, sprouted crackers, raw nut trail mix, coconut chips, raw veggies, and dried fruit.

The condiments I enjoy are limited to mustard and grass-fed butter. My salad dressing is olive oil based with lemon juice, spices and/or apple cider vinegar. I sweeten my desserts with stevia, coconut sugar, maple syrup, and molasses. I flavor my meals with sea salt, and fresh or dried spices.

Since I changed my diet I no longer suffer from GERD. I don't restrict acidic foods that once irritated my bladder. The constant burning in my genital area is gone! My irritable bowel and chronic constipation have resolved now that eat so much fiber. I eat foods that I was allergic to such as almonds, avocado, cabbage, and eggs. Once I consistently ate healthy foods all my symptoms magically disappeared!

Healing Insight 12: Your inner child needs you.

Teal Swan, *Overcoming the Past: Trauma, the Shadow, and the Inner Child* podcast compliments of Hay House Radio

This insight has proven to me how necessary it is to foster, nurture, and care for that inner child. Your inner child must heal before you can heal. We don't realize that trauma we have experienced or perceived as a child can haunt us for the rest of our lives. Teal Swan made it very clear that the trauma did not have to be as severe as physical or sexual abuse. Just the fact that our inner child perceived it as a trauma of maybe feeling abandoned, feeling alone, feeling unsafe or afraid is enough to keep us stuck. She explains this in her podcast, *Overcoming the Past: Trauma, the Shadow, and the Inner Child*, compliments of Hay House Radio.

It is enough to keep us attracting the same types of situations in our life. I know that may be hard to grasp but the Law of Attraction is a real law in science just like the Law of Gravity. Please remember, you must process and release emotion not serving you. This is necessary so that you can stop having the same thoughts, feeling the same way, having the same experiences, and reliving the same events from your past.

One activity I did was to create a timeline. The instructions were to start at age five and list any events or memories in five-year increments, to create a list of items to meditate 'Tap' on. My first memory was of me refusing to eat spinach. I remember how slimy and smelly the canned spinach was. Yuck! I ate everything else on my plate hoping I could slide by. No luck. My mother insisted I eat the spinach. My dad naturally agreed with my mother. So, I sat there in front of my plate. My two brothers ate their spinach and were excused from the table. But there I was as stubborn as an ox. I didn't give in, and neither did my mother. I sat at the table for two hours after dinnertime. I can still feel the ice-cold stares my mother gave me as she would walk by to check on my progress. She would say, "The sooner you eat it, the sooner you can get off your chair." Still, I refused.

I felt the anger, resentment, and frustration build. But still, I just couldn't eat that spinach. It was slimy, cold, it smelled, and it made me nauseous. Even though I knew I was disappointing my mother I just couldn't make myself do it. I really wasn't trying to be defiant. I wasn't trying to piss her off or make her look stupid in front of my dad and brothers. I was sincerely grossed out by the spinach on my plate. I'm sure I expressed all of that to my mother which probably made things worse. That's why I was still sitting there.

It seemed like an eternity. The temperature in the room seemed to drop with the cold stares and the silence between us. I remember thinking, *I just want my mom to love me. I just want to be a good girl.* I felt sad but this stupid spinach was standing in the way of pleasing my mother. My brothers would pass by the kitchen. They would look at me like *oh s*** you're going to be in so much trouble!* Their eyes had pity. At the same time, I could feel that my dad was tense. He went and sat in the living room to watch TV. He was so serious. I just kept thinking, *I wonder what Dad thinks of me? He's probably mad at me too! How am I going to get out of this?*

I could feel the hard chair on my bottom as I sat there. I tried to be comfortable. I was falling asleep at the table when my father finally declared, "That's enough of this, you're done, get off the table and go to bed." I believe I was six when this incident took place. I often wondered if this spinach incident was the reason the relationship between my mother and I never flourished. I wonder if my mother looks back on this as the first time that I defied her. The first time that I challenged her. The first time that I made her feel so angry at me. I wonder if she just could never get over it and held it against me.

Those are the thoughts I had so many times throughout my life. Those are the feelings I have felt that have made my heart ache so many times. The funny thing is that I actually love spinach now. I eat it several times a week! No, I don't buy canned spinach, only fresh spinach. But every time I eat my spinach I think about that incident and I say, "Look, Mom, I'm eating my spinach, aren't you so proud of me?" This is just the first of many incidents that I had unprocessed emotions around related to the relationship with my mother. Throughout my life, there were many more incidents, more severe, with more hurtful words and actions between us.

All of these incidents and events were listed on my timeline. Yes, I have meditated 'Tapped' on every one of them, many of them multiple times. By releasing the emotion that was connected to all of these incidents throughout my life, I have been able to see the beauty. All the love and all the caring moments that my mother and I shared. Nick Ortner explains it like this: "Tapping clears away what's been blocking you from seeing all the good that happened during a certain memory." So, if for no other reason, please 'Tap' on these events and memories from your childhood to honor your inner child. Process and release any thoughts, emotions, events, or memories to let go. Allow yourself to see all the good that has been and is in your life right now!

'Tapping' also known as Emotional Freedom Techniques (EFT)

"Tapping meditation is one of the four ways to change your programs," according to Dr. Bruce Lipton. He explains, "The four ways are hypnosis, repetition, energy psychology (which EFT 'Tapping' is considered) and high-impact events such as traumatizing life-changing events that make us realize we need or want to change like a near-death experience or having a terminal illness."

'Tapping' is a meditation technique that stimulates acupressure points to help you release emotion. 'Tapping' simply sends signals to calm the area of the brain that controls the stress response. The amygdala is the part of the brain that causes the stress response and releases stress hormones like cortisol and adrenaline when you feel threatened. This self-defense mechanism is wonderful when you are truly threatened but when your body stays stuck in this self-defense mode it is extremely detrimental to your mind, body, soul, and spirit.

There are nine basic acupressure points that are usually stimulated during the Tapping Meditation Process. However, to simplify this process you will only stimulate the collarbone point. It is located two inches below the collarbone on each side. This acupressure point will be stimulated 'Tapped on' for the duration of this Tapping Meditation.

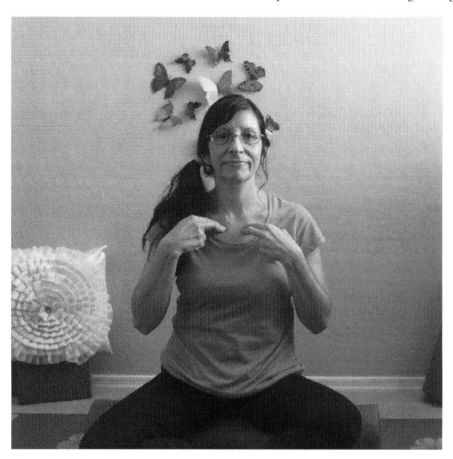

Collar bone acupressure point.

The basic structure of 'Tapping' is to start with acceptance and truth about what is bothering you. Use statements that express exactly how you feel, what you think, what you're experiencing, or what you've experienced in the past. Remember when you hold on to the past it keeps you stuck; that is what is causing this physical, emotional, or spiritual pain.

The second step in 'Tapping' is to process and release. 'Tapping' works by helping you to release those emotions, those thoughts, those events in your life that you are holding on to which cause physical, emotional, and spiritual pain. Over time, this pain robs you of your energy and depletes your ability to love, heal, and forgive. This pain torments you every second of every minute of every hour of every day of your life!

The third step is to renew positive energy by 'Tapping' on feelings of hope, healing, and peace. This is where the healing begins! Once you finally process those emotions, thoughts, and events that are holding you back, your mind, body, soul, and spirit are in sync. Now your (parasympathetic) nervous system is primed for healing.

Activity:

"Shhh!"

Instructions:

- Think of one phrase you tell yourself daily.

- Example: I'm so stupid, I can't heal, I'm broke, etc.

- Use this phrase to guide you to know how to quiet your critical voice.

- Write this phrase below and rate how high your level of judgment is on a scale of 1-10.

Daily Challenge:

Turn Hope into Action!

"Tap & Release!"

'Tap' on each phrase that is not serving you to release negative thoughts. Use *The Tapping Meditation to Release Negative Thoughts* script (below).

Welcome to *The Tapping Meditation to Release Negative Thoughts*.

This is Deborah Lucero from liveyourfulllife.com. In this Tapping Meditation, we will focus on releasing negative thoughts.

You can pick one acupressure point to stimulate or start on the eyebrow point and move through as you repeat the statements out loud or to yourself. If you do move through the points please remember to include Spirit Gate 7 located on the side of the wrist. You can choose to close your eyes to add an extra level of relaxation and comfort to this technique.

Find a place where you feel comfortable.

To begin we will take three deep breaths to calm the central nervous system. Breathe through your nose, exhale through your mouth. We will do that again, breathe in and exhale through your mouth. One last time, breathe in and exhale through your mouth. Begin 'Tapping,' at your own pace.

Karate chop: Even though I tell myself (insert phrase), I choose to forgive myself and honor how I feel.

Karate chop: Even though I tell myself (insert phrase), I choose to forgive myself and honor how I feel.

Karate chop: Even though I tell myself (insert phrase), I choose to forgive myself and honor how I feel.

Eyebrow: All of this judgment, I feel it in my body, mind, soul, and spirit.

Side of the eye: I have this judgment because I don't know how to be my own friend.

Under the eye: I only know how to judge myself because I have done this my entire life.

Under the nose: How can I ever get rid of this judgment, if that's what my old programs tell me to do?

Under the chin: I judge myself so harshly every day because it's just a habit.

Collarbone: How can I be gentle with myself?

Under the arm: Everyone else around me judges me too.

Side of the wrist: I just want to figure out how to let go of this judgment!

Top of the head: What if I could just release some of this judgment?

Eyebrow: I choose to forgive myself for not knowing how to be my own friend.

Side of the eye: I choose to change the habit of judging myself daily.

Under the eye: I choose to stop judging myself so harshly.

Under the nose: I choose to stop thinking, (insert phrase).

Under the chin: I choose to take responsibility for my emotional well-being.

Collarbone: I realize it is up to me to learn to be my own friend.

Side of the wrist: I'm releasing this judgment, so I can be kind to myself.

Under the arm: I'm releasing this judgment, so I can create a space to heal.

Top of the head: I am releasing all of this judgment right now from my mind, body, soul, and spirit.

Take a deep breath. Release any feelings, thoughts, and events holding you back right now. Slowly open your eyes when you are ready.

You may feel the need to do more 'Tapping.' If so, please measure your level of judgment on a scale of 1-10 before and after each round of 'Tapping' until you feel relief. A number below five is a good stopping point.

From everyone here at Live Your Full Life, may you find hope, healing, and peace!

Healing Insight 13: Every time you were sick you were told you had to go to the doctor.

Biology of Belief, Dr. Bruce Lipton

When I read *Biology of Belief* by Dr. Bruce Lipton, I thought about this healing insight, and I wondered, *What does it really imply?* That if you need help, you seek out a doctor? Or is there an underlying message that you are helpless? You cannot help yourself so you must go to the doctor every time you are sick? In some instances, going to the doctor may be necessary, but what are we telling our bodies when the first thought we have is *I'm sick and the only way I'm going to feel better is if I go to the doctor?* We're telling our bodies that we have no control, that we have no part in our health. No role and no responsibilities. We are giving up our power to heal without even knowing it. We are releasing our ability to even think of a solution to help ourselves.

This false belief that we are sick so we must go to the doctor plays a huge role in the lack of self-care that we should give ourselves. I do remember my mom saying, "You have to take care of number one because no one else will take care of you." But I didn't hear this until after I was overworked, stressed, and my health was declining. Where were the lessons to teach us that we are worthy of taking care of ourselves? We are valuable as human beings, and it's okay to take care of ourselves.

We do a decent job of feeding ourselves, putting ourselves to bed at night, making sure we have showers and brushing our teeth. I'm not talking about that. I'm talking about our minds, our souls, and our spirits. We were never taught to clear out those negative thoughts. We were never taught to release those emotions that were keeping us stuck. We were never taught to help our souls, or our spirits feel whole. Feel connected to a higher power for the purpose of taking care of ourselves. We were taught that every time we were sick, we had to go to the doctor. We were also taught that every time we were sick we had to take a pill. This chain reaction of thoughts caused us to become dependent on outside resources to help us rather than relying on our own ability to heal.

This was a major obstacle for me because I relied on this process for as long as I can remember. I would say to myself, "I feel sick; I need to go to the doctor, so I can feel better." As soon as I went to the doctor, I did feel better. Sometimes the doctor didn't even give me anything. But just because I thought that my healing had to come from seeing the doctor that's what I made myself believe. I could not start feeling better until after I had seen the doctor. I had to physically go to the doctor.

I know this sounds trivial. Take a moment to process the action involved. You're having the thought that you are sick, and you need to see the doctor, so you can feel better. Then you feel that to be true so you take action. You get yourself up. You get yourself to the doctor. You tell the doctor what's going on and then magically you start feeling better.

What if you could use that process to heal yourself without going to the doctor, without needing the medications? What if you could use functional medicine and alternative treatment instead of a pill to feel better? This never even occurred to me to be an option. I always thought one pill is good so more pills are better. That's what I felt to be true, and that's what I acted upon. I ended up being on 18 prescription medications all with overlapping or multiple side effects causing me to have more symptoms than when

I started. Those side effects included nausea, dizziness, constipation, irritability, aggression, fatigue, numbness, depression, and the list goes on.

Even though I came from an educational background as an occupational therapy assistant—it was my job to teach people how to be functional, how to use alternative types of treatment, and to help them alleviate their symptoms—I was not applying it effectively to my life. Yes, I used a heating pad when my muscles ached but only after I had already taken pain medication or a muscle relaxant. I was not doing any preventive treatment either. I remember two different occasions so vividly, where this was brought to my attention. I was doing my first round of pelvic floor therapy after I had bladder repair surgery. I had gone back to work, and my sciatica was raging. Not to mention my pelvic floor was in excruciating pain.

I told my therapist, "I use my ice pack when I drive to keep my sciatica from flaring up." He said, "Well that's a good start but have you ever thought of actually changing position every 30 minutes to prevent the pain altogether?" He went on to explain, "If you can pull over on the side of the road, get out and stretch or walk around for a couple of minutes, that is what you really need. Because then you won't have the compression on your sciatic nerve and then you won't need that ice pack." Wow! I felt stupid. But I was grateful he pointed this out to me. So that's what I tried to do especially when we traveled a long distance.

Another incident I remember so clearly was when I was hoping to remove antacids from my medication list. I was still trying to help my liver heal. I told my primary physician that I was going to start cutting back the dosage. He said, "Why don't you just prevent heartburn altogether? Try this, eat a big breakfast, eat a lighter lunch, and eat a small dinner, especially with very little meat because it is the meat that is causing the most issues. The meat is what needs more acid to be broken down. If you do this, you won't need your antacids." Epiphany, right? That's exactly what I did and bam, it worked! I wonder sometimes why I didn't get this information sooner. Why didn't I ask? Did my doctor think I didn't want to know?

Doctors are used to giving out pills. I have found that if I ask a physician or any medical provider gives me ideas for alternative treatment or natural treatments they are very open to offering those treatments. So, remember, even if you do still have the thought in your mind that when you get sick you have to go to the doctor, don't just think that you have to go for a pill. Try asking for some alternative treatment ideas or preventive ideas instead. This will help you to start detoxing your mind from old programs and detox your body from the toxins of medication.

Healing Insight 14: Souls never die. Love never dies. It is our responsibility to cleanse our energy every day and to protect it.

Hay House U Live 2017 Conference, James Van Praagh

This healing insight is especially close to my heart. I have lost several of my immediate family, sooner than I would have liked to. Starting with my father in 1994, his death was especially difficult for me because I was Daddy's girl. It took me 20-plus years to process the death of my father. To release the sadness, the sorrow, and the grief that was in my heart. It wasn't until April of 2017 that I had the honor of meeting James Van Praagh at the Hay House U Live 2017 Conference. My youngest son and I volunteered for the Hay House work program. We were assigned to work with Mr. Van Praagh on Saturday. The first words from his mouth that morning touched my soul.

He said, "Souls never die. Love never dies. It is our responsibility to cleanse our energy every day and to protect it." Just the way that he expressed himself, I felt his emotion in every fiber of my being. I had believed for so many years that death was final. Death seemed so difficult to process because of the fact that you may never see your loved ones again. Sadness, sorrow, and grief had consumed me too many times. If I just had this insight even ten years earlier, I think it could have saved me from sinking into the deep wounding sadness that I felt when I lost my maternal grandmother in September of 2012.

This was the beginning of the end of my health. My grandmother was my rock. I was totally crushed when she passed, three days before I was scheduled for my bladder repair surgery. My family and I were headed to see her when I received the call that she had passed. We were at the gas station filling up. Her funeral services were two days after my surgery. So, I never got any closure because I was unable to attend the funeral due to travel restrictions from my surgery.

I remember when the father made his rounds at the hospital the morning after my surgery. He asked if he could pray for me. I wanted so badly to ask him to pray for my grandmother's soul. But I knew that if I spoke I would break down. So, I just nodded yes. Maybe that's why this healing insight is so close to my heart because I have carried around so much sadness, sorrow, and grief that it seemed to heal me that day in April. It helped me realize that I was not losing my family members forever. Their love and souls never died; only their bodies were gone.

An equally important message of this insight is that it is our responsibility to cleanse our energy field every day and protect it. This cleansing is to help us process and release thoughts, emotions, events, and memories that are not serving us. Protecting our energy field helps to keep our energy strong and flowing freely. Once our energy gets stuck in any part of our body, we become stuck to our past. When this emotion is stuck, in our bodies our health begins to break down, causing us physical, emotional, and spiritual pain. Mr. Van Praagh also made it very clear that you must first cleanse your energy and then protect it. If you just protect it and you don't cleanse it, then you are keeping all of the thoughts, emotions, events, and memories that are not serving you stuck. This made total sense to me. I knew I had to apply this healing insight to my own daily life.

In November 2013, Del, a very close friend of mine, gifted me a chiropractic session to try acupuncture. I had never been to a chiropractor. I had mixed emotions due to my mother and father's beliefs. My mother was for chiropractic care, and my father was against it. I never really knew what my belief was. I was a bit worried. I guess because I was in so much pain, but I figured I couldn't get any worse. So, I made the appointment.

As the doctor inserted the needles, he asked me, "So what event caused your illness?" I didn't hesitate because I knew. I said, "It was the death of my grandmother last September." He must have written that in my file, because when the nurse came in to chat with me she said, "When you're ready to process all of that emotion from that event, let us know how we can help." Sadly, that was the first and last appointment I had with that particular chiropractor. Mostly for financial reasons. But I also think it was because I just didn't know how to begin the process of healing my mind, body, soul, and spirit.

Healing Points to Treasure

1. Hope will inspire you to take action, to fight back from any situation. Self-care does make a difference.

2. Your thoughts cause feelings and your feelings cause changes in your body. Whether those changes are positive or negative depends on your thoughts.

3. Know your triggers. 'Tap' during stressful situations. 'Tapping' simply sends signals to calm the area of the brain that controls the stress response.

4. Toxic relationships have to go. Write a 'Thank-You List' and 'Tap' to find the hope, the healing, and the peace.

5. You have two minds, the conscious and the subconscious mind. When you journal, the conscious mind creates the plan, and the subconscious mind carries it out.

6. Explore new techniques, treatments, or remedies to feel empowered. Take responsibility for your health and self-care. Believe it or not, you are worth it!

7. You can't expect change without changing your BS story. The Law of Attraction is as real as the Law of Gravity! Think a positive thought, send out the positive energy, and feel the emotions of how that thought would feel if it were already a reality.

8. Most of the habits that are being run by your subconscious mind 95% of the day are bad habits. 80% of your thoughts are negative every day! Also 98% of the time you are having the same exact thoughts that you had the day before.

9. Realize what type of energy is in your environment. Evaluate how it is affecting you and how you are affecting others. To achieve homeostasis, a state of balance and well-being, you must nurture your body, mind, soul, and spirit in every sense of the environment.

10. The stress center part of the brain (amygdala) stores aggression, joy, sadness, and fear. 'Tapping' is a coping skill to process and release emotions not serving you, and a tool to change your old programs.

11. Evaluate what you put into your body. Not just food, but thoughts in your mind. Feelings you are storing in your heart and brain. Events holding you back from healing. I can't stress enough how the process of healing must include your mind, body, soul, and spirit! I hope you will remember that.

12. Your inner child must heal before you can heal. Realize trauma you experienced or perceived as a child can haunt you for the rest of your life. Process and release emotions not serving you. This is necessary to stop having the same thoughts, feeling the same way, having the same experiences, and reliving the same events from your past.

13. The false belief, 'every time you are sick you have to go to the doctor,' plays a huge role in the lack of self-care that you should give yourself. You are giving up your power to heal without even knowing it. Start detoxing your mind from old programs and detox your body from the toxins of medication.

14. 'Souls never die. Love never dies. It is your responsibility to cleanse your energy every day and to protect it.' Once your energy gets stuck in any part of your body, you become stuck in your past. Your body and your health begin to break down causing you physical, emotional, and spiritual pain.

CHAPTER TWO

Step 2 Releasing Emotion: Healing Insights 15–28

Use Emotional Freedom Techniques (Tapping Meditation) to access the process of super learning to push the record button on the subconscious mind to fully process and release what is not serving you!

I didn't understand what was keeping me stuck, making me sick, and robbing me of my energy. The answers were right under my nose but because I was trapped in the stress response cycle, I wasn't able or willing to look deeper. I kept ignoring obvious signs that I needed to nurture my entire being. I needed to accept the reality that I was both the problem and the solution!

What I was about to learn about releasing emotion would free me of unhealthy thoughts and emotions. I was reliving events and memories that were steering right back to the same experiences every day. I ignored my body. I tormented my mind with negative thoughts. I hated myself and who I had become. I shamed my spirit by not realizing that I needed to nurture myself—until my health crashed! Finally, I realized I needed to embrace my body, forgive my mind, love my soul, and honor my spirit.

I cannot stress enough how important it is for you to find the source of your physical, emotional, and spiritual pain. This chapter will help you dig deep, foster your emotional well-being, and nurture your mind, body, soul, and spirit. Then and only then will you be able to process and release thoughts, emotions, events, and memories not serving you.

'Tapping' is an amazing healing technique that will allow you to forgive yourself as well as others. It has the power to change false beliefs and old programs to release you from your most painful experiences. It will help you to take back your health, to take control of your life, to find relief today!

Healing Insight 15: I am enough!

Nick Ortner, *I'm Not Enough,* Tapping Meditation

I still didn't think I was good enough. I had so much guilt, shame, anger, resentment, sadness, sorrow, grief, and heartache. I had so many emotions around the loss of multiple family members, my financial burdens, and from the relationship with my mother. The Tapping Meditation that Nick Ortner wrote, *I'm Not Enough,* made my tears flow. It made me experience all of the emotion of every memory associated with it. I thought, damn, this sucks. This is hard work. I can't do this.

I had always been a tough girl. I was the Enforcer, the disciplinarian parent. I had been on my own since I was sixteen. I was a teen mom. My husband (then boyfriend) and I chose to move out and get a place together when our oldest son was about three months old. From that day forward I had been in survival mode. I worked part time while I was still finishing high school. I was always independent. I wasn't going to let myself down. I wasn't going to let anyone else down, either. I pushed myself even in my teens. I went against doctor's orders to stay out for six weeks. I rested very little even the two weeks that I was home after delivering my son.

My maternal grandmother advised me to stay in bed and take care of myself. My son was born in December. She said, "The cold is going to hurt you. You need to wrap your belly and stay inside." I didn't listen. I was living at home with my parents at the time. My husband was living with his parents, also. We wanted to show off the baby. So, we went visiting everyone instead of having them come to see the new baby.

Two weeks after I returned to school, four weeks after my son was born, I ended up with an infection. But I still didn't listen. I just took the antibiotics. I went back to school because I didn't want to get behind. I still didn't want to show that I was weak. I obviously didn't learn self-care early on despite my grandmother pleading with me. I look back and see that I repeated this pattern throughout my life.

I always stuffed my emotions down. There was always this incident or that incident. So, I just tried to block it out. I didn't necessarily remain silent. I was definitely the one to call out my mother and stand my ground when I felt that I or someone I loved was hurt by her.

It wasn't that I was not expressing my thoughts, my emotions, and my beliefs. The fact was, I was not processing and releasing all of this garbage that was piling up. I still felt the same emotions I did the day I refused to eat my spinach. Things didn't get any better during the process of making funeral arrangements for my father. My mom and I were butting heads yet again. As outspoken as I am, I called her out once again over the phone. Of course, the conversation ended with a click.

That conversation haunted me for years. How could I love myself when I don't feel love? Honestly, I think I felt this even before we had that conversation. I believe that is why I never chose to take care of myself, to love myself and to nurture myself. I didn't feel worthy of love, acceptance, or forgiveness, not even from myself. But because of this healing insight and consistent use of the Tapping Meditation technique that has all changed. I finally realized 'I am enough!'

Tapping Meditation has taught me that you must love, accept, and forgive yourself in order to be loved, accepted, and forgiven. You must improve your self-worth as a human being. You are worthy by default. What a concept! It totally blew my mind. It was not what I had pounded into my head, not anything close to what I had applied to my life. I am thankful that I have learned the process of releasing thoughts, emotions, and memories not serving me.

That is why my 5-Step Process includes detox, releasing emotion, mindset, reprogramming your mind, and exercise/physical activity. I'm hoping to show you that you are worthy by just being alive! You are deserving of health, wealth, love, and happiness! It is within your ability to create the life you deserve! It is your responsibility to honor your mind, body, soul, and spirit!

Activity:

Health, Wealth, Love & Happiness Review

- Let's take a deeper look at our lives.

Instructions:

- For each category decide if you feel "I'm Not Enough" or "I Am Enough."

- Then list 3 reasons why you feel that way.

Health, Wealth, Love & Happiness Review – Activity Sheet

Category	I'm Not Enough	I Am Enough
Health		
Wealth		
Love		
Happiness		

Daily Challenge:

Turn Hope into Action!

Tapping Makes It All Better!

- Pick one category from the Health, Wealth, Love & Happiness Review activity that could be better.

- Go back to Healing Insight 12 and use the Tapping Meditation to release negative thoughts.

- Please take responsibility for your own emotional well-being.

- Allow yourself to process and release any and all thoughts, emotions, events, or memories that are not serving you today!

Remember we are looking for action! We want you to start creating these habits that are going to be healthy in your life. You have to take action today! That's how you make it happen.

Healing Insight 16: Forgiveness is the gift you give yourself.

The Power of Your Subconscious Mind, Dr. Joseph Murphy

This has been a powerful healing insight for me. I always knew that forgiveness was crucial to healing any pain. But I didn't know how to apply it to my life. That's why the book, *The Power of Your Subconscious Mind* by Joseph Murphy, changed my life forever! I didn't have an understanding of the process of forgiveness. I thought I had to be face-to-face with the person I had hurt, or that had hurt me, in order to forgive myself, or that person. There are so many different ways that I have learned to forgive throughout this journey of self-development.

Just by knowing that I could forgive someone without being face-to-face with them was uplifting. That meant I didn't have to deal with any drama. I didn't have to butt heads. I didn't have to explain myself. I didn't have to defend myself. I could simply forgive that person or even forgive myself for hurting someone. I could process the emotions around it and reap the benefits of forgiveness which are so crucial to the process of healing your mind, body, soul, and spirit. I had so many memories and so many incidents that needed forgiveness.

I didn't even realize that I could forgive myself. I thought I had to carry the guilt. Somehow, I thought the punishment of being guilty would keep me from being mean again. Saying mean things and doing mean things. Or reacting in a horrible way. But it didn't. All the guilt and shame did was keep me trapped. I was chained to the physical, emotional, and spiritual pain that I so desperately needed to be freed from. To begin my journey of healing, I had to learn to forgive. As I mentioned in The 5-Step Process For Fibromyalgia Relief course, you must honor your mind, body, soul, and spirit.

Here are several methods to apply the process of forgiveness to your life. First, think of someone that you need to forgive. Make a list of positive things that person has done for you. Another way to forgive someone is to record the incident and the emotions that are holding you back on a piece of paper. Then either burn it or tear it up into shreds to let it go forever! Still another way is to write a forgiveness letter or forgiveness note so that you can make it real and lasting. Remember, the process of physically writing things down is very similar to meditation. So, the added benefits are worth the time.

Another simple way is to actually write a gratitude letter and list everything that you are grateful for. List everything that you have learned from this person. List everything that they have given you. I'm not talking about physical items. I'm talking about love, support, forgiveness, honesty, loyalty, and the list goes on. Then you take this to the next level, which is to read the letter of gratitude to that person, personally. This will allow you to bathe yourself in those emotions, so you can feel that gratitude. This process also lets you see how your gratitude touches and changes you as well as the other person. You're probably saying that's crazy, right? That's exactly what I said until I did it.

I have used all of these methods to help me forgive myself and others. I have allowed myself to open up to myself and with others to be able to heal. I want to show you different levels or different ways that you can implement the process of forgiveness into your life. Whatever your level of comfort is you can pick and choose; whatever method works best for you and for a certain situation. I remember how healing it was to write the list of wonderful memories or things that my mother had given me throughout my life. I remember how freeing it was to write down some of those false beliefs and hurts that I needed to forgive myself for. To just watch them burn or to have them torn up into shreds and be done with them forever was liberating. It was so cleansing, so healing, so empowering. I remember when I wrote a forgiveness note to myself and how touched I was. I needed this gentle caring love for myself to move forward.

Another deeply touching method was a gratitude letter I wrote my husband. I thought about it for several days. Finally, I just wrote it. Believe me, writing this letter was the easy part; reading it to him was not so easy. I remember telling him that morning, "I have something I need to read you. My gratitude activity was to write a gratitude letter and then read it to the person I wrote it to." I asked him, "Can I read it to you?" He just said, "Sure." It took me a while to start reading because of all the emotion surrounding this letter. I also had to pause throughout the letter so I wouldn't totally break down and cry.

Even though it was one of the most difficult activities that I have completed during this self-development process, it has been one of the most healing. It was so important for me to express to my husband my gratitude for his unconditional love throughout our marriage. I needed for him to know that I appreciated the fact that he could still love me. No matter how horribly I had behaved. No matter what I did. How I acted. Or what I said. I was grateful that he was still able to love me, unconditionally. This gratitude activity also made me realize the lesson that I was learning from my husband being in this life. I don't think I had ever truly realized that he was teaching me the blessing of unconditional love until I wrote that letter.

I hope you will find some of these methods helpful. I want to help you learn to allow yourself to open up, so you can process and release thoughts, emotions, and memories not serving you. Please find it in your heart to forgive yourself. Once you do, you will be able to forgive others also. When you apply the process of forgiveness to your life, you will create a space to heal. So please remember forgiveness is the gift you give yourself.

Healing Insight 17: I believe you.

Dr. McRae, Health First Medicine

This healing insight came at such a tender time along my journey. It was still early on when I was trying to process and release so much emotion and memories from my past. It was a time when I hadn't even yet realized that I was stuck and trapped by these unprocessed thoughts, emotions, and memories. I didn't understand that's what was causing my pain. I hadn't yet made the connection that my pain was psychosomatic. It was related to my psychological state of being.

I remember being at my doctor's office trying to explain the multiple symptoms that I was experiencing. I vented to him about the never-ending pain that I had around the clock. Not really knowing why I was experiencing it or how to help myself. I told my doctor, "Sometimes I think people don't really understand or believe that I'm so ill or that I'm in so much pain." I thought this way because I had continued to maintain my grooming throughout this time, even though I felt so bad.

I went on to explain to him that I had discussed this to some level with a PA that I used to see at a different doctor's office. I also mentioned the fact that the PA had suggested to me that I should continue to keep up my grooming because it would help me to keep moving forward, even though I was in so much pain. But I almost felt like it was a double-edged sword. I felt like it was causing my medical providers to overlook my symptoms and my pain. I wondered if they were just seeing that I had showered, that I had combed, and that I had taken the time to apply makeup. I thought maybe they didn't believe me despite how I described that I was extremely fatigued, in severe pain, and weak.

I also went on to tell my doctor that I never liked drama. There was plenty of that throughout my life. For this reason, I tried to keep my reactions subtle. I wondered if this was making my medical providers question my condition. His response to me was, "I believe you." Those three words touched my heart, my soul, and my spirit that day. I felt the sincerity and the tenderness of his acceptance. I felt his desire to truly help me find a solution to all of my symptoms and pain. I realized that my emotional and spiritual being needed this validation. I realized that I could share my symptoms and my pain with my doctor. I didn't have to convince him. I could allow him to guide me to a solution, so I could find relief.

I know a doctor's main purpose is to prescribe medication, but I have found through this process that if you simply ask for an alternative method or some guidance, doctors are very willing to share what has worked for them. Or what has worked for other patients. They will share alternative treatment resources that are available. I felt so relieved when my doctor told me, "I believe you." I didn't feel like I had to keep convincing him. I could simply report what was going on in my body and he would accept it at face value. That is exactly what he did.

I share this healing insight with you because I know your symptoms. I feel your pain. I know how frustrating it is to describe your symptoms and have someone make you feel like you are making it up. Or make you feel like you are exaggerating. Believe me, no one can make up the misery involved in fibromyalgia and all the related medical conditions that come along with it. I know your physical, emotional, and spiritual pain. I know the pain of feeling like you have lost everything.

You are not alone. I know it feels that way. Please remember, there are five million Americans living with fibromyalgia. That is too many people living in misery. That is so many people fighting to take their health back. That is so many people trying to control their life. My goal is to help you recognize that you are important! Your thoughts and your emotions matter! You have the ability to take your power back! You can fight fibromyalgia! I want to help you find relief today!

Healing Insight 18: How are you feeling?

Ezekiel Lucero, my youngest son

This healing insight is from my youngest son. No matter what day of the week or how I feel my youngest son always asks me, "How are you feeling?" Even if he's at work, he'll text me on his break just to see how I'm feeling. I didn't realize how important this was to my healing. In the beginning, I even used to get bugged when he would ask me because I felt so crappy. Also, I am not one to lie or cover things up. So, I'm sure that I was blunt and not as polite as I should have been. I did tame my answers after a while so I didn't feel like I was lying to him or anyone else and especially not to myself. I would at least say, "I'm okay" or "mostly better."

This healing insight goes back to the fact that we need to realize we are cared for and we are loved. It is difficult for our family members to see us in a situation of not being 100%. Especially when we are living with a chronic condition that wears and tears on us daily, day in and day out, around the clock. This bit of sincerity can go a long way. The biggest benefit of this healing insight is the thoughts that you think. They become feelings and feelings take action and action shows up as changes in your body.

So, remember to ask yourself, "What am I telling my body?" If someone asks you how you are feeling, of course, you don't want to lie. But you want to focus on the most positive statement that you possibly can make. That way when all of the cells in your body are listening, and they are, your response will be heard as the positive energy that you are circulating with this statement. It's so easy to get caught up in speaking exactly how we feel. But focusing on it too much in a negative way just plays into our need to complain.

How does the saying go? "Misery loves company." You complain then the person you are talking to complains. Then before you know it it's just a cycle of negative energy going back and forth. Try to say the truth of how you're feeling but then move on. Reframe your response to be positive. You will be doing yourself a favor by staying out of this negative cycle of feelings, thoughts, actions, and changes in your body. I know this sounds silly, but if you can interrupt those thoughts you will get yourself thinking in a positive state of mind. Your thoughts will become feelings of gratitude. That gratitude will help you take action. Those changes will take place in your body. You will begin to feel better.

Remember, people really don't want to hear you complain and they do want to know how you are feeling. So, try to rephrase anything that might sound like a complaint. Also add a bit of inspiration, hope, or peace that you have found that day. Even if you have to really dig deep to find the positive, there is always something good that has come from every day that we live.

The more often you choose to focus on the positive, the more grateful you will stay. The more you stay grateful, the more grateful you will actually feel. The more grateful you actually feel, the more great things you will bring into your life. Then you can make great changes in your mind, body, soul, and spirit. If all else fails, and you really just need to vent, don't feel guilty. Just do some 'Super Tapping.' That is when you vent and 'Tap' while you are expressing what needs to be processed and released.

Remember, when you process and release your thoughts, emotions, and memories you begin to heal. That's exactly the purpose of this healing insight. It is to help you realize that you can create a life you deserve. Please know that I am trying to inspire you to feel the hope, the healing, and the peace. I know that physical, emotional, and spiritual pain are real. I am not trying to make light of it, in any way. I have been there, stuck in that pain, wondering how even the next second much less the next day could be better. So please honor how you feel and express it so that you can create a space to heal! Then you can live a full life!

Healing Insight 19: Stress makes us reactive, not responsible.

The 7 Habits of Highly Effective People, Stephen R. Covey

Stress keeps you from being able to think clearly, to problem solve, and to be resourceful. I was so reactive for the majority of my life I didn't even realize that there was a difference between reacting and responding. Reacting is part of the stress response cycle. You're unable to have a proper response. It's just that simple. Reacting keeps you in the state of victimization. You feel like everyone is always trying to offend you. Everything seems to be targeted towards you. Everything feels like an insult. You wonder what you did to deserve this.

Reacting to a situation is purely a habit. It just happens because that's what you do when you're in the stress response cycle. You try to protect yourself. Then you end up offending other people, targeting other people, judging other people, and blaming other people. Being in the stress response cycle goes right along with being a victim. This partnership of reacting and feeling like a victim is a match made in hell! It keeps you trapped from realizing that you actually have a choice to control your emotions. You can actually choose how you respond, to a situation. You may not be able to choose or control how someone else reacts or responds. But you always have the choice, the opportunity to choose how you respond, how you control your emotions. You cannot be hurt if you do not perceive that someone has hurt you.

It is that simple. The situation probably was not directed at you. It was just that you were reacting as a defense mechanism. Overreacting takes place most of the time once you get stuck in this pattern. I lived my life for too long, too many years reacting, blaming, judging, feeling victimized, and not knowing any better. How could I change when I didn't even know what needed to be changed? Stephen R. Covey described the term 'responsible' in his book, *The 7 Habits of Highly Effective People,* as being 'response-able.' In other words, you are able to respond.

Wow! I felt so dumb again. I thought, *What have I been doing all my life? Was I always this 'duh'? Or was it just truly the stress response cycle that was making me act this way, since I had been stuck in it for so long?* I was reacting like an animal trying to survive every situation. I thought I was threatened, when most of the time, probably 90% of the time, things weren't even directed at me. I perceived every incident as a big deal.

The main point I want to make here is that I am hoping you can realize that the stress response cycle is so damaging to you when you are stuck in it for a long period of time. The stress response cycle really does keep you trapped. From knowing, from using your mind, from using your intelligence, from using your compassion, from using your kindness, from using your better judgment. It keeps you from expressing your love.

The stress response cycle keeps you from realizing you are not a victim. It also keeps you from knowing that you are 'response-able' to create your own life. You are 'response-able' to create a life that is full of health, wealth, love, and happiness. You have the ability to create a life that is bathed in joy, gratitude, and freedom from physical, emotional, and spiritual pain. You can design a life that is truly abundant. You're probably thinking, okay, now I know what the definition of responsible is, but how do I reach that state of mind at this moment?

Whatever you're doing, whatever you're thinking, whatever you're feeling, whatever pain might be in your mind, body, soul, or spirit, please start 'Tapping' two inches below your collarbone. You don't have to say anything. You don't have to do anything other than just 'Tap.' Just be in this present moment while you're listening to my voice. Continue to 'Tap.' 'Tapping' on an acupressure point will send a signal to the stress response center in your brain. It will help your brain to know that it is okay to be calm, that you are safe; because you truly are safe.

'Tapping' will help you flush out the aggression, the fear, and the sadness stored in the amygdala (the stress response center of the brain). 'Tapping' will help you to feel the joy that is stored there as well. The 'Tapping' that you're doing is creating a space for you to heal right now, at this moment! You don't have to wait until tomorrow. You are healing right now! So please choose to be 'response-able.' Choose to leave the stress response cycle behind. Choose to stop reacting. Choose to start making those changes in your life that you are capable of. Choose to find the hope, the healing, and the peace that this technique will give you; so you can maximize for a full life!

When you're ready you can stop 'Tapping'. Take a deep breath and release any and all thoughts, emotions, and events or memories that are not serving you right now.

Healing Insight 20: The 5 Love Languages

The Five Love Languages, Gary Chapman

Pam Kays was one of my pelvic floor physical therapists. During one therapy session, we were talking about our significant others and how they seemed to change over the years. She asked me, "Have you ever read the book, *The Five Love Languages*?" I responded, "No, what is it about?" I was very curious. She went on to explain that the author Gary Chapman had discovered that there are five love languages.

We all have our own specific love language. Because that is our love language that is also how we express our love to others. When we love others through our own love language we may not be giving others the love that they need. We may not be speaking their love language. This is the basic concept. Wow, this freaking blew my mind! Seriously, I had never heard of this. *Where have I been, in a cave?* Yes, basically, I had been stuck in my cave brain! In a stress response cycle for too long.

I had heard of personality styles or characteristic traits, but never love languages. I was so curious that I went straight to the library and rented the audiobook. Once again, I convinced my husband to listen to this with me just as I had convinced him to do the Tapping Solution Webinar with me. The concept was amazing!

The author had decades of experience in marriage counseling. He had identified the five love languages as: words of affirmation, acts of service, gift giving, quality time, and physical touch. You will have to read the book to figure out what love language you are as well as your significant other. It is not uncommon for people to have a primary and a secondary love language. So, for instance, my primary love language is acts of service. My secondary love language is quality time. So of course, I just absolutely love it when someone pitches in and gives me a hand hence the word acts of service. That's when I feel totally loved. I also like to spend quality time together. When I can spend time with someone, I feel extra special! This was all starting to make sense to me. I needed this at least two decades ago!

I also saw where this could be tricky. Because whatever love language you are is the love language that you typically speaking to others. So, I tend to show my love by doing acts of service for others by helping. I also find myself expressing my love by spending some of my time with others. This is great for me because they're my love languages, but what about my husband? Those are not his love languages. So, I am not expressing love to him the way he understands and vice versa. His love languages are different from mine. He's loving me and showing me love the way he likes to be loved. We were totally not communicating with one another appropriately.

Once I was finished with the book, I wondered how we were still together. I decided to do the six-month activity. Honestly, my marriage had been strained for several years, even before my health totally crashed. This book was heaven sent because I needed a clue. I needed a fresh start. I needed hope that there was some guidance, a plan, a blueprint to follow. I have learned so much on this journey. Sometimes I'm embarrassed to say how amazed and dumbfounded I had been when I discovered this new information that should have been available to me years ago!

I urge you to read the book! Listen to the audiobook, whatever it takes! Discover what your love language is. Discover what your significant other's love language is. The author has even written books about using this concept if you're single, or to find your children's love language, or to figure out how to be successful at work by communicating with your co-workers using their love language. It makes so much sense. Pick up the book or rent the audiobook today and find out what your love language is!

This healing insight will help you find hope and purpose in your marriage. It will help you realize that you're not just butting your head up against a brick wall. There is a process involved. There is a way to speak clearly to the needs of your significant other and to receive the love that you are yearning for. Learning to speak your significant other's love language is easier than you think because the author has listed so many examples, activities, tips, and ways that you can learn to do this. He knows that you naturally speak your own love language as an expression of your love to others. So, he provides this extra support to help you be successful.

Bonus insight: Did you know that love is the highest emotion you can feel? It is that higher-level emotion that Dr. Joe Dispenza speaks of. You must feel higher-level emotions such as acceptance, service, joy, peace, and love to connect your thoughts to your feelings and feelings to your actions. Your actions will make your thoughts and feelings become a reality because of your positive energy. This will automatically cause positive results (changes) in your body, and in your life. Remember, even in your personal relationships, you are sending out positive or negative energy. The energy you send out is the energy you get back. So, please take the time to look up this resource. It's a wonderful, beautiful resource that you deserve to have!

Healing Insight 21: Our emotions are making us sick.

Functional Health Summit, Dr. Axe

When I heard this healing insight from Dr. Axe I sat on my yoga mat totally in awe! I could not believe what I had just heard. Even though I had never heard this before, it made total sense with what was going on in my life. I thought about all of the stress and the emotions around what I had been bottling up and carrying around for decades. As I thought about the events in my life and all the emotion, I realized that it was no wonder my body had crashed. I was just wondering how my body had even lasted as long as it did with all of the emotion that I had never processed and released.

I didn't have a coping skill in place besides crying and praying. As I thought about it even more, I could see the connection between emotions and illness. When my body started falling apart in 2010, we had decided to move back to Colorado to be closer to family again. It was not the wisest choice. We only lasted six months and moved back in February of 2011.

This was during the recession. My husband didn't find work the entire six months we were in Colorado. He didn't find work for another six months after we moved back. Our finances were a burden, and I thought I could handle it by just taking on more clients. I eventually added more hours at work, until I was working twelve hours a day. I was gone fourteen hours a day with the drive time. Proof of my emotion being connected to illness was very apparent in November of 2011 through February of 2012. I had three sinus infections in four months. Then my bladder started acting up. I thought I was just having an overactive bladder and UTI symptoms.

By March of 2012, I realized my body was taking a hit and I could no longer remain in the same position working that many hours a day. So, I changed jobs. My health continued to decline. I had blood in my urine. I was diagnosed with interstitial cystitis in July of 2012. By September of 2012, I had a bladder repair surgery. As I mentioned before, my grandmother passed away three days before that surgery was scheduled. So, I was unable to attend her funeral. All of that stress, sadness, sorrow, and grief just kept compounding my health conditions—making things worse!

I knew by January 2013, when I returned to work after that surgery, that I could no longer fulfill my duties. I was having difficulty keeping myself safe and keeping the children that I worked with safe. At the time, I was working in a private day school for children with severe behavioral and developmental disabilities. Initially, my thought was just to cut my hours. But I still had to finish the school year. My reduced caseload wouldn't start until late summer.

As I looked back to the periods in my life where I had been so stressed, I began to notice that there was an illness that came right along with it. It was amazing how clear the evidence was supporting this insight! I thought to myself, wow, I have suffered for no reason! If only I would have known to process and release all of these emotions I have been holding back for all these years, maybe I would not have had to suffer so much. If I only had a way to do that. Maybe I wouldn't have needed half of the surgeries that I have had. Maybe I wouldn't have tortured my body so much without even realizing it. I still had to sit and soak up this information.

Even though I could see the evidence, it was overwhelming to realize that my illness could have been prevented. Yes, Dr. Axe was absolutely correct! It is our emotions that are making us sick. I'm so glad that I received this healing insight when I did. Even though my health had already declined so much, it was uplifting to know that if I could just process and release this emotion, then maybe I could start feeling better. That was the best news I had heard in a long time! I was grateful that I had started to understand, more and more, what Dr. Axe was trying to share with his message! Now I had this new ammunition to fight back. I was ready to take back my health, take control of my life, and find relief! Thank you, Dr. Axe!

Healing Insight 22: It's not your job to change others; you can only love them.

"Surrogate" Tapping Meditation, Jessica Ortner

This is one of the hardest insights for me because I am a perfectionist. I am hard on myself as well as others. I always want to have some type of control over the situation. If something is working for me, I want to share it with others. I want them to gain the benefits that I am gaining. I want them to make changes that I know will be beneficial in their life. That will improve their health. That will help them to find the peace they deserve.

I have butted heads the most with my husband over this because I know how much of a worrier he is. I know now, but I didn't realize it then. I couldn't even see it in my own life. I know now how much stress he had. I know how long he had been in that stress response cycle, right along with me. I realize how it had affected his life, health, and energy as well.

I didn't always feel like I was trying to change him. I felt as if I was just trying to show him a better way. I know that he has to want to make these changes in his life. I cannot make him take action even though I think he should. I have had to 'Tap' on this insight many times because I had to release my need to control. I had to release my need to judge. I had to release my need to want to overly influence my husband's decisions.

The best thing to do is to just love your family, support them, help them, guide them, and keep from pushing them. When you push too hard, you just get pushed back! It doesn't solve anything. It just creates more conflict, more stress, and a never-ending cycle of negative energy. You end up with more emotions to process and release. So please find it in your heart to realize that no matter what your best intentions are, they can only be put into action in your own life. You cannot make someone implement even the best of habits into their own life if they are not ready.

The 7 Habits of Highly Effective People, by Stephen R. Covey, made another connection for me. I realized what he meant by using your 'circle of influence'. It simply means that within your circle of family and friends you can have a positive influence on them without overstepping your boundaries. What a simple concept. This made so much more sense than what I had been doing. It was still somewhat difficult for me to apply this concept to my life. I had to learn to listen, try not to give advice, and just keep my healthy lifestyle changes consistent.

Sometimes, I feel that these healing insights are heaven sent and perfectly timed. They seem to enter into my life exactly when I need some guidance, when I need some hope, when I need some faith, and when I need some support. Remember, "When we shine in the darkness, it allows others to shine as well," Jessica Ortner. She knew exactly what she was talking about. I'm sure that is why she included this healing insight in her Surrogate Tapping Meditation.

Don't get discouraged, just know that your perseverance, your consistency, your strength, your hope, your faith, your love, and your support does make a difference. Your positive energy is being felt all around you. You are making those connections between your thoughts and your emotions. By taking action, you are sending out positive energy for a positive life to become a reality. Keep moving forward, and you will begin to see that others around you will start noticing the changes in your life. They will want what you have. They will start asking, "What are you doing? Can you please teach me?" This is all possible when you can feel the hope, the healing, and the peace!

Healing Insight 23: Why you so mad?

Siana Lucero, my granddaughter

My granddaughter is now 5 and a half. She has been very aware of my emotions since she was old enough to talk. I have been working on releasing anger from my life since 2014. Even up until about March of 2017, I have had moments of difficulty. Please know that these techniques don't mean you will never feel another emotion. We are human. We have to feel emotion.

Emotion is just emotion even if people label it negative or positive. We still have to experience these emotions. There are times to be sad, to be angry, lonely; there are times to be calm. There is a time for every emotion like the song *Turn, Turn, Turn* by The Byrds. I love the last line of the song: "A time for peace, I swear it's not too late." I feel as if it were written specifically for me. :)

Feeling the emotion is not the problem. The problem is when we do not process and release these emotions. When we stay stuck in the stress response cycle. So, when my granddaughter asked me in March, "Why you so mad, Nana?" it broke my heart. I have been working so hard at this. I have been trying to improve.

Before, my granddaughter would ask me, "Are you mad?" or "You mad, Nana?" I would explain to her, "No honey, I'm not mad. I'm frustrated, I'm tired, I need a break, or I'm hurting." Whatever the reason was I would try to explain it to her. But this time she didn't ask me if I was mad, she knew I was mad. That day, I made a promise to myself that I would never let her feel my anger again.

I looked back at my childhood, and I thought of my grandparents. I spent a great deal of time with my maternal grandmother and my step-grandfather. My grandmother was like my mother. I never remember her giving me that feeling that she was mad. I know there were times when she was upset. But I never felt that raw anger from my grandmother.

I didn't want to keep letting my granddaughter feel that raw anger from me. I had been working so hard to keep my emotions in check, especially my anger. I've been trying hard to watch my triggers, to know when I need a break ahead of time. I try and take deep breaths and do a little bit of yoga or find time to do some Tapping Meditations.

I want to give my granddaughter the programs that she needs. I want to show her that it is okay to do a one-minute meditation. It's okay to 'Tap.' I want to teach her these coping skills that I didn't learn. I don't want to pass on my old programs. I don't want to teach her how to stay in the stress response cycle. I want to help her to know that yes, you will feel emotion, but you must process and release it. I owe that to her, to my own children, and to myself. I want them to feel the hope, the healing, and the peace.

Healing Insight 24: We have to feed our systems with emotional well-being.

Truth About Cancer Summit 2015, Ard Pisa, Author, Researcher & Speaker

This healing insight is something that I picked up from the Truth About Cancer Summit in 2015. I learned so much from this free online event. It was amazing to realize that so much illness is caused by lack of self-care, as well as misinformation provided by the medical community. I am just so grateful that there are people like Ty Bollinger, the founder of Truth About Cancer, who is brave enough to ask the hard questions. This healing insight stuck with me because, at the time, I was working so hard on my own emotional well-being.

It seems like we do a decent job of taking care of our physical bodies and that's about it. We sleep, we eat, we bathe, and those are all physical needs. But what about our emotional well-being? As children, many of us are taught that we are not supposed to cry. We are not supposed to express our emotions because we will be thought of as weak. I grew up around several boys, so I was a tomboy and I toughed things out. This has served me well, at times, but it also has been something that made me think I had to hold in my emotion and just 'take it'.

I mentioned this to my pain specialist during the injection that I believe triggered the week-long migraine that I ended up with in May of 2014. The doctor asked me what part of the country I was from because I chose not to go under anesthesia. I told him I was from the Southwest and that I did grow up by some farms, but I did not grow up on a farm. He said, "I thought you were from the Midwest because usually, that is where the tough farm girls are from." He just laughed and said that usually, the little petite women are the tough ones who handled this kind of procedure without anesthesia. I told him that I had always toughed things out throughout my life but that I wasn't sure if it was really to my benefit. He laughed again and continued with the procedure.

I want to take a look at this a little more deeply because our mindset is what causes us to think a certain way, to feel a certain way, and to act a certain way. Be aware of that. So you don't get into situations where you're unable to process and release your emotions. I believe what Ard Pisa—author, researcher, and guest speaker for Truth About Cancer—was trying to say with this healing insight is that it is okay for us to be tender to nurture our souls and our spirit. It is okay to take time to honor ourselves. To listen to what our soul is telling us that it needs.

Take time to connect with your spirit, your true self, so that you can live that truth each and every day, instead of living in the mindset of old programs that we don't even realize are not serving us. The best way that I have found to apply this healing insight to my life was to become my own friend. I didn't even know this was an option until I started following Nick Ortner and his sister Jessica Ortner from TheTappingSolution.com.

This concept was quite shocking to me since I had been beating myself up all these years. Telling myself that I had to be tough. That I had to suck it up and I had to grow a tough skin and just deal with it. But this is exactly the opposite of what I really needed to be doing for myself. I can't even explain it fully. How wonderful it is to take time to nurture myself emotionally and spiritually connect. This is a part of my day that I really treasure!

These are the feelings that I have when I am connecting with spirit. I feel safe. I feel comfort. I feel secure. I feel protected. I feel love and forgiveness, as well as my own self-love and self-forgiveness. I feel humbled. I feel empowered. I feel grateful. I feel thankful. I feel blessed. I feel connected. I feel whole. I feel such unity with the universe. I believe this is what Ard Pisa meant by 'feeding ourselves emotional well-being.' So, take the time to nurture yourself emotionally and connect with spirit. It is a beautiful way to honor your mind, body, soul, and spirit. So please do it.

Healing Insight 25: Remember who loves you!

Deborah Lucero

This healing insight initially came to me when I attended my cousin's husband's funeral in April of 2016. Then I experienced another level of this healing insight a year later in April of 2017. You might remember I had cut ties and isolated myself from my mother's family. I didn't want them to be involved in all the drama. So, when I learned of my cousin's loss, I didn't even think about attending the funeral. I just figured I would be there in spirit. Since I had learned the 'Tapping' acupressure point to release sadness, sorrow, and grief (which had helped me process my father's death that same year) I told my husband, "I think I need to go and teach Vangie the 'Tapping Point' for sadness, sorrow, and grief." So that's what I did.

Even though it was a funeral, it was a family reunion for me. I hadn't seen any of my mother's family since 2005 when my brother and my grandfather passed away, within a week of each other. I felt so much love, so much acceptance, so much forgiveness, so much understanding, so much joy and so much peace. I was truly in heaven. I actually had fun. We laughed. We joked. We cried. We prayed. We hugged. It was so nice to reconnect with all of my family again.

Did you know, research has proven that when you see people that you know, your brain releases dopamine, the happiness hormone? Maybe that explains why I was so happy. Whatever it was, I benefited from this visit so much. I explained to them why I had kept my distance. I realized that I loved and missed them just as much as they loved and missed me. That trip made me realize that I had stayed away too long. There was no tension at all. Also, since my husband didn't go with me, I was able to give my family my full attention.

During the Hay House U Live 2017 conference, I experienced this healing insight again during a meditation exercise guided by James Van Praagh. I had a memory that came through so crisp and vivid in my mind. I know that this memory has been there in my heart forever, but because I had all of the pain surrounding the relationship with my mother, I was never able to access that memory until that day. This memory was about the time when my mother gave me permission to plant sunflowers seeds along the sidewalk of our front yard. We didn't have a very big yard, but she gave me the go-ahead anyway.

In my memory, it was early morning probably before school. I was standing on the sidewalk facing my sunflowers. I could see my parents standing on the porch, and my brothers were standing behind me. We were in awe of the beauty of the sunflowers. We were in disbelief of how much the sunflowers had grown. Not only did I see this memory, but I found such wonderful emotions with it. I could feel the love, the pride, and the acceptance. Not just from my father, but from my mother as well. I felt all that love, the pride, and the acceptance that had been there since I was a child. It felt as warm as the sun's rays in my memory.

This memory warmed my heart. I wanted to stay there forever, in the beauty of that memory. I was so touched. I didn't feel anger, resentment, hate, sadness, sorrow, grief, shame, or guilt. None of those emotions were there that day. It was all pure love and acceptance. The joy was so overwhelming; I couldn't wait to share this memory with my husband and sons when we met for lunch. I described in detail everything that I was able to see and feel in that memory. I was delighted! Because I had actually felt on this day like all of this hard work that I have been doing on this journey of self-development to heal my body, mind, soul, and spirit had actually come full circle. I felt as if finally, I was more conscious than I ever thought possible. I was more in control of every aspect of my life than I ever knew I could be.

I was more connected to myself on every level. I felt so connected to my soul family. This is what I call all of my deceased family now. I also felt more connected to my soul community. This is what I call all of my mentors; all of the great thought leaders that I follow. I was more connected to my true self, to spirit. It was truly a time of pure joy and enlightenment.

Please take the time and do the work. It may not be easy, but it is definitely worth it! Process and release the emotions not serving you. Then you can have access to all the beautiful memories and all the wonderful blessings that surround you. Enjoy the time you have to reconnect. Feel how rejuvenating this is to your mind, body, soul, and spirit!

Healing Insight 26: Unconditional Love

Alex Lucero, my husband

I often wonder what lessons I am meant to learn while I am here on earth, especially now that I am on this journey to live a full life. I understand that even though we have challenges we can learn a powerful lesson. As I look back on my entire life, I have realized how much unconditional love I have been blessed with right from the beginning. I had unconditional love from my father, my grandmother, my step-grandfather, my paternal grandparents, my brothers, and my extended family. Now I realize that I even had unconditional love from my mother. I have realized just lately that one of the greatest gifts of my marriage has been the unconditional love of my husband.

As I mentioned to you in another healing insight, I wrote a gratitude letter to him based on his unconditional love for me. I would love to share that letter with you, but I'm not sure if he would give me his permission. Even if I did get his permission, I don't know if I could read it without totally breaking down. So much of what I wrote in that letter was about some of the most difficult times in my life, some of the most painful and some of the weakest times of my life, as well. Since I 'toughed it out' the majority of my life, I think it kept me from even visiting the idea of what lessons, true lessons I could learn. It kept me from the exceptional blessings I had already received in my life because I was focused so much on the negative.

Also, I was focused on the pain, the hurt, the heartache, the sadness, the sorrow, and the grief not to mention the anger, the resentment, the shame, and the guilt. I couldn't focus on the love, the unconditional love, the joy, the peace, the happiness, the strength, the faith, the courage, the hope that I was showered with my entire life. It's so amazing that once you process and release emotions not serving you, how much beauty truly lies beneath the surface of the pain and the heartache. The anger had been blinding me from seeing how blessed I was and how blessed I am.

Take a moment and look back at your life. Just think of what lessons are buried within the challenges of your life. Maybe it's unconditional love, patience, acceptance, or forgiveness. Whatever it is my hope is that you will take it to the next level. That you will allow yourself to process and release these emotions that keep you stuck from seeing the countless blessings you have been unable to see and appreciate. Please know that this process may not be an easy one. You must do the work to process and release all that you have been holding in and holding on to for a lifetime. But know that when you do you are opening yourself up to a wonderful new way of living.

Not just a new way of thinking but a new way of being. A new way of perceiving. You are allowing yourself to see the possibilities. You are allowing yourself to choose to appreciate all of the good things that you have going on right now in your life. You are allowing yourself and giving yourself permission to know that it's okay to process and release emotions. It's okay to be gentle. It's okay to have this awareness of what is beyond our everyday lives. It is okay to be present, truly present in the moment, to be conscious, to use your conscious mind in a way that will benefit your mind, body, soul, and spirit.

You can create a space to heal! You can move forward in your life and create a new mindset, a mindset that belongs to you, a mindset free of false beliefs, a mindset free of doubt, a mindset free of programs that don't belong to you. This is your time! This is your life! The possibilities are endless! Remember every possibility is available. You just have to observe it so it can become a reality.

I know at times it may seem like I'm repeating myself or it may seem like I'm going off on a tangent and that it's not related. But it is! It is all related! We are a whole being and because of that, we must nurture every part of our being. This is a totally new way of thinking! I understand that, but it is a fact even if it seems so abstract and so out of reach. You can attain it! The most exciting part of creating the 70-Day Course is to share with you all of these healing insights! To give you the matter-of-fact, concrete proof that you are capable of creating the life you deserve! You just have to know how to maximize for a full life. This is how you do it!

Healing Insight 27: Wisdom is having a memory without experiencing the emotion.

Tony Robbins

This is another great healing insight that I was blessed to learn from Tony Robbins! It has been another challenging healing insight for me. Because I have had such an emotional connection to so many memories and experiences in my life as I learn to process and release emotions not serving me, I understood exactly what Tony Robbins is saying. I can now look back on my childhood at some of those most painful memories and see that there was so much more than pain. There was so much more than anger and resentment.

Once you have processed and released emotions not serving you, they no longer have power over you. This is where the wisdom comes in. Now you can go back and think about that memory, and the emotional charge is gone. This allows you to see the situation with a more neutral set of eyes. This gives you the opportunity to realize lessons that need to be learned. It lets you experience all the good that was always there, and you just couldn't see it because you were so controlled by your emotions.

One of my most painful memories was when I refused to eat canned spinach; I discussed this memory in Healing Insight 12. I have thought of this memory so many times in my life because of the control it had over me emotionally. It kept me stuck in the past. I still wondered if my mother was angry at me and resented me for challenging her. I have 'Tapped' on this memory and the emotions surrounding it multiple times.

You are probably wondering what the wisdom is that I have been able to take from this memory. I now am able to see the pure love my mother had for me. She was trying desperately to teach me how to eat healthy by reinforcing that I had to eat my spinach. This memory has also shown me that I had emotional strength even as a child. This is apparent because I stood my ground. I believe my mother was actually proud of me for this, because it is one of her best traits. I am also glad that she taught me how to take a stand.

This situation showed me that I had unconditional love from the beginning. It confirmed the fact that my mother loved me, unconditionally. It confirmed that she loved me no matter what. It pointed to the reality that no matter what I did, what I said, how I acted, I was still worthy of her love. I had been searching for her love my entire life and there it was buried in this memory. Because I had been experiencing emotions of anger and resentment I perceived this memory as a trauma.

Had I not experienced this situation so early in my life, I might have missed out on all the hidden blessings. Whether I like to admit it or not this situation gave me one of my greatest qualities. I have been able to use this strength throughout my life. I didn't realize it, but this is probably the biggest reason I am here writing this book right now. This strength has allowed me to fight back against fibromyalgia and all the other ailments.

I hope I have made it clear to you that there is wisdom to draw from even in your most painful memories. The lack of knowledge and the perception of being in distress have blocked you from recognizing these beautiful lessons. Your past does not have to haunt you. Your emotions do not have to control you. My wish is that I can help you learn how to process and release the emotions holding you back from living a pain-free life and loving every minute of it. Take a stand with me and fight!

Healing Insight 28: Emotions are not attached to you, so why are you attached to them?

Quantum Enigma, Bruce Rosenblum and Fred Kuttner

In the book *Quantum Enigma*, Bruce Rosenblum and Fred Kuttner describe when Albert Einstein compared our attachment to emotions to our attachment to furniture. Einstein said, "The furniture is not attached to you, just like an emotion is not attached to you." He asked, "So why are you attached to them?" According to Dr. Joe Dispenza, emotions help you realize and identify with who you are. It is not your soul or your spirit that needs an identity, but your ego. It is your physical being that keeps you stuck to your emotions.

Another reason you are attached to these emotions is because there are memories or events that are associated with them. Dr. Dispenza cautions, "Where you focus your attention is where you place your energy." When your emotions keep you stuck in the past or daydreaming about the future, you miss out on the present moment. You are stuck in the physical realm, having difficulty releasing emotions around past thoughts and events. Or you are perseverating and thinking about future events that you don't know how to make a reality.

When you are attached to emotions that have crippled you from being your true self, these emotions make you re-experience the entire trauma that was associated with them. The brain doesn't know the difference between the past, present, or future. Wherever you are focusing your attention is where your brain keeps you. The problem with this is that you experience these emotions as if the event is taking place at the moment you are thinking about it. If your emotions keep you connected to an event in your past that you were angry about, your body will release stress hormones. Your brain thinks it needs to protect you, so it keeps you in the stress response cycle. You stay stuck in this cycle because you were not taught how to process and release these emotions so you can be in the present moment.

If you are eager to create a space to heal, to create a life that you deserve, you must realize that this insight has such a strong message! You must apply this healing insight to your life. This healing insight leads back to processing and releasing these emotions. That is because emotions really do truly keep you stuck. You remain stuck in the past and you remain stuck wondering how you are going to achieve the future. You never place your focus on the present so that you can turn your aspirations into reality.

Dr. Joe Dispenza explains, "We just keep placing our past on to our future." You never get into the flow of being present, so you can be the creator of an amazing life.

I hope this healing insight helps you focus on how to be present. I hope you understand that emotions are not attached to you—so you don't need to be attached to emotions. I trust that you will recognize that it is okay to let go of the past. It is okay to stop being focused on the future. It is perfectly fine to focus on today. In fact, today is the only time that really matters. It's the only time you have access to. The past is gone, and the future may never be.

Can you imagine what you could accomplish if you remained conscious more than 5% of the day? This healing insight took my level of understanding to another dimension. It made me realize why I had been stuck and couldn't move forward. Know that you can use the Tapping Meditation Process to free yourself from these emotions. Next, you can use the Law of Attraction to focus on the positive and be grateful, so you can live in the present moment. Then you can create the life you want! Because now you are truly present to take action to propel yourself forward.

The most important fact of all: the only time you are able to create is when you are present! So please focus on being present. Focus on what you can do today! Don't beat yourself up for what you did in the past. For what you can't change. Let It Go! Stop focusing on the future because you may never see the future. Use what you have learned and take action! You do have the ability to create your own life. Make this the best day that you can. Make it a great day because today is a brand-new, never-lived-in day! Create this day with your heart's desire!

Activity:

"Let It Go!"

Instructions:

- List an emotion under each category.

- List an event related to each emotion.

- Pick 1 emotion and the related event.

- Use this simple Tapping Meditation Script below & Let It Go!

"Let It Go!" Activity Sheet

	Past	Present	Future
Emotion			
Event			

Let It Go Tapping Meditation Script

This is Deborah Lucero from liveyourfulllife.com. In this Tapping Meditation, we will focus on an emotion and an event that needs to be processed and released so you can let it go.

You can pick one acupressure point to stimulate or start on the eyebrow point and move through as you repeat the statements out loud or to yourself. If you do move through the points please remember to include Spirit Gate 7 (located on the side of the wrist). You can choose to close your eyes to add an extra level of relaxation and comfort to this technique.

Find a place where you feel comfortable and safe.

To begin we will take three deep breaths to calm the central nervous system. Breathe through your nose, exhale through your mouth. We will do that again, breathe in and exhale through your mouth. One last time, breathe in and exhale through your mouth. Begin 'Tapping' at your own pace.

Even though I feel_____(emotion)_____I honor how I feel and choose to let it go.

Even though I feel_____(emotion)_____I choose to move forward and let it go.

Even though I feel_____(emotion)_____I've been stuck too long so I choose to let it go.

I feel this_____(emotion)_____but I'm the only person still hurting so I choose to let it go.

I'm tired of this_____(emotion)_____making me sick and I choose to let it go.

This_____(event)_____still feels so wrong, but I choose to let it go.

This_____(event)_____should have never happened, but I need to let it go.

This_____(event)_____has taken away so much of my energy so I choose to let it go.

This_____(event)_____has made me feel this way for way too long so I choose to let it go.

This_____(event)_____is over and I choose to let it go.

Take a deep breath. Release any feelings, thoughts, and events holding you back right now. Slowly open your eyes when you are ready.

You may feel the need to do more 'Tapping.' If so, please measure your level of resistance on a scale of 1-10 before and after each round of 'Tapping' until you feel relief. A number below five is a good stopping point.

From everyone here at Live Your Full Life, may you find the hope, the healing, and the peace!

Healing Points to Treasure

1.   You must improve your self-worth! You are deserving of health, wealth, love, and happiness! It is within your ability to create a life that you deserve! It is your responsibility to honor your mind, body, soul, and spirit!

2.   Forgiveness is crucial to healing any pain. You don't have to be face-to-face with the person you hurt or the person that hurt you in order to forgive. Find it in your heart to forgive yourself.

3.   You are important! Your thoughts and your emotions matter! The sincerity and the tenderness of acceptance are necessary. Your emotional and spiritual being need this validation.

4.   Ask, "What am I telling my body?" All the cells in your body are listening. Interrupt negative thoughts to get in a positive state of mind. Your thoughts will become feelings of gratitude. That gratitude will help you take action.

5.   The stress response cycle keeps you from realizing you are not a victim. This partnership of reacting and feeling like a victim is a match made in hell! You have a choice to control your emotions. You are 'response-able' to create your own life.

6.   There are five basic profiles to express love. Whatever profile you are is the way you express your love to others. Figure out your profile as well as others to receive and express love appropriately in all your relationships.

7.   See the connection between emotions and illness. Illness can be prevented. 'Tapping' is a great coping skill to process and release emotions that are making you sick.

8.   The best thing to do is love your family, support them, help them, guide them, and keep from pushing them. When you push too hard, you get pushed back! It creates more conflict, more stress, and a never-ending cycle of negative energy.

9.   Feeling the emotion is not the problem. The problem is when you do not process and release these emotions.

10.   Your mindset is what causes you to think a certain way, to feel a certain way, and to act a certain way. Be aware of that. Take the time to nurture yourself emotionally and connect with spirit. It is a beautiful way to honor your mind, body, soul, and spirit.

11.   Remember who loves you. Process and release the emotions not serving you, so you can access all the beautiful memories and all the wonderful blessings that surround you.

12.   Choose to appreciate all the good things you have going on right now in your life. It is okay to be present, to be conscious, to benefit your mind, body, soul, and spirit.

13.   There is wisdom to draw from your most painful memories. The lack of knowledge and the perception of being in distress have blocked you from recognizing these beautiful lessons. Your past does not have to haunt you. Your emotions do not have to control you.

14.   When your emotions keep you stuck in the past or daydreaming about the future, you miss out on the present moment. The only time you are able to create is when you are present!

CHAPTER THREE

Step 3 Mindset: Healing Insights 29–42

Use an abundant mindset to free yourself from being in a chronic stress response cycle. Listen to what your body needs. Listen to your soul to know what emotions need to be processed and released from your mind. Listen to your spirit; to live your truth, your purpose, and realize your full potential!

I didn't know different types of mindsets existed. I didn't realize that I inherited a scarcity mindset rather than an abundant mindset. I wasn't blessed to learn the concept of the Law of Attraction. I didn't get this basic message from anything I was taught in school. It definitely was not something you learned in the workforce. This message just wasn't there!

What I was about to learn about mindset blew me away! Sure, there were guidelines for exercise and a healthy diet. What about your soul? What about your spirit? What about your mind, your thoughts, and your feelings? What about your emotions? What about all those events that keep you frozen in time? That prevent you from realizing you are a beautiful being and you are worthy of health, wealth, love, and happiness?

This chapter will teach you how to harness the power of the Law of Attraction by creating a positive mindset. You will learn how powerful your thoughts really are! You will understand how the brain and body function, so you can use this knowledge to your advantage. You will discover how to allow others to help you along the way. You will also realize that you have what it takes! Yes, you can have it all! You don't have to suffer! You don't have to sacrifice! You can find this balance. You can have a full life! It is possible!

Healing Insight 29: Know the Law of Attraction?

Alex TRI Lucero, my oldest son

As I mentioned in The 5-Step Process For Fibromyalgia Relief course, my oldest son TRI was especially supportive and helped me to realize that I needed to learn what the Law of Attraction was. He knew that I was focusing on the negative. He knew that all of the emotions I was feeling had me stuck and in pain. He knew that my body was stuck in the stress response cycle. He realized that all of the stress hormones were being excreted and causing me to stay stuck in the cycle of negativity, and I was bringing misery into my life.

He didn't want to offend me, so in his subtle way, he just asked me if I knew what the Law of Attraction was. Of course I didn't but when I Googled it, it was an insight that has changed my life forever! Don't get me wrong, at first, I thought, what a crock. Easy for that to be applied when your life is running smoothly, right? I thought, *What about when your life is a mess? When you're in constant pain; when you have such a brain fog and such stress that you can't even make a rational decision?*

The Law of Attraction has the power to make us all the creators of our own destiny. Yet somehow, this simple process was not so easy for me to implement into my life. But little by little, with all the other techniques, remedies, and alternative methods that I was using, I was able to get the ball rolling. I can't forget to mention how 'Tapping' has helped me to be able to apply this healing insight to my life. By being able to process and release emotions not serving me, I was able to have more control over my thoughts and not be so reactive to situations in my environment.

By implementing physical activity, like light yoga and stretches, I was able to ease some of my physical pain. Which also helped me gain even more of my thought process back. By cleaning up my diet and making those changes part of my new healthy lifestyle I was feeling even less pain and clearer with every bite of nutritious food. The vitamins and supplements that I added to my daily regimen were helping me to improve the severe vitamin D deficiency, iron deficiency, relieve body aches, and boost my energy. These vitamins and supplements eventually replaced medications, which gave me even more access to my thoughts.

Taking action and learning self-care was a must. Also helped me feel more in control, not only of my body, but of my life. So gradually, the positivity was starting to flow. I was starting to learn that these emotions were holding me back. I realized these emotions were making me sick and were robbing me of the life I once knew. These emotions were keeping from the even better life that I never knew I was able to have. I was beginning to be able to interrupt those negative thoughts. I was learning to use my critical voice. To know what I needed to 'Tap on.' The more I listened to my critical voice without judgment, the more I was able to have the mental power I needed. The more I listened to the aches and pains in my body and nurtured myself. The more my body responded in a positive way.

I was feeling inspired! I was thinking more clearly, thinking and seeing the possibilities as well as feeling empowered! I was feeling alive! I was taking action, and I was taking notes! I was seeing the changes in my body and the changes in my life! I was noticing how this positive Law of Attraction cycle was working for me! I was realizing that this basic concept was a huge piece of knowledge that I should have been taught as a child. It should be taught to every child. It should be part of every educational institution. It should be standard core curriculum in my opinion. Imagine how healthy, how happy, how loving, how fulfilled we could be as a society if we had been taught this one insight!

Imagine how you could be living your purpose. How you could be connected to your true self. How you could be living the life that you choose to live not a life that was programmed into your mind. Not a life of pleasing others because you didn't know better. Not a life of misery because you were not taught how to nurture your mind, body, soul, and spirit. Please take the time to understand what the Law of Attraction is. I advise you to realize that the Law of Attraction is a real law, just as the Law of Gravity is. I am hopeful that you will use this healing insight to the benefit of your own well-being. I urge you to teach your children and your grandchildren about this. They can create a life that they deserve! They too can maximize for a full life!

Activity:

"Observe Your Thoughts!"

"You are not your thoughts; you are the observer of your thoughts."

~Oprah Winfrey~

Instructions:

- Set a timer for 3 minutes.

- Sit and observe your thoughts.

- Listen to your thoughts and list them under the categories.

"Observe Your Thoughts!" Activity Sheet

Positive Thoughts	Negative Thoughts

Daily Challenge:

Turn Hope into Action!

"Clear Your Mind!"

- Be proactive! Use this list of activities as preventive care!

- Clear your mind daily!

- These activities are not just for when you're feeling bad!

- Use these activities to live a full life today!

"Clear Your Mind!" Check List

✓ Tapping Meditation

✓ Exercise

✓ Eat Healthy

✓ Quiet Your Critical Voice

I wanted to share my Daily Vitamin/Supplement List with you.

My Daily Vitamin/Supplement List

Vitamin D 1,000 IU	7 tablets daily (joint health/dietary supplement)
Calcium 220 mg & Vitamin D 200 mg	1 tablet daily (bone health/dietary supplement)
Magnesium 250 mg	1 tablet 2x daily (nerve & muscle health/ dietary supplement)

Iron 65 mg 325 mg Ferrous Sulfate	1 tablet daily (general wellness/dietary supplement)
Multi Vit/plus 18 mg iron/400 IU vitamin D 400mg folic acid /6mcg vit B 12	1 tablet daily (general wellness/dietary supplement)
Vitamin B12 60 mcg	1 tablet daily (heart & nerve health/ dietary supplement)
Fish Oil 1000 mg	1 tablet 3 x daily (anti-inflammatory/ dietary supplement
Vitamin E 400 IU	1 tablet daily (breast health/dietary supplement)
Aloe Vera 25 mg	1 tablet daily (bladder health/dietary supplement)
Zinc 15 30 mg	1 tablet daily (immune health dietary supplement)

Healing Insight 30: You just have to know the next step!

Nick Ortner, *The Tapping Solution*

This healing insight helped me take back my health, take control of my life, and find relief. It also helped me to create The 5-Step Process For Fibromyalgia Relief course as well as develop the Healing Insights 70-Day Course. Eventually, because of this healing insight and many others, I was able to create a plan. A thought, one simple thought. Feel how it would feel if it were a reality and allow my subconscious mind to carry it out, so that I could make the changes I wanted in my life. So I could live the life I wanted. So I could have a wholesome balance of health, wealth, love, and happiness.

I must mention that Tai Lopez's *67 Steps* helped me realize what characteristics were getting in my way. The main one that I discovered was analysis paralysis. I am great at creating plans. I'm actually very good at follow through. But sometimes I just analyze things to death. That keeps me stuck. It keeps me from taking action.

Again, my perfectionist mind was getting in my way and keeping me from realizing that I just needed to get started. I just needed to take action! I just needed to know what the next step was, that's all. Just as Nick Ortner knew what he wanted to achieve; he took it step by step. I knew that I wanted to take back my health, my life, and I wanted pain relief.

We make our decisions either from fear or love; as James Van Praagh says, this can be either to your advantage or to your disadvantage depending on which emotion you are making those decisions from. As I look back, too many times, I made decisions from fear because I was in the survival emotions of anger which includes fear. Remember when we start experiencing one survival emotion, it's a package deal. The snowball just gets bigger.

You're probably wondering, "How do you stop that from happening or how do you reverse it when it's already in full force?" You just have to know the next step. You have to stop yourself. You have to find yourself in this process. You have to clear your mind. Clear your emotions and take action. That is why journaling is so beneficial. It helps you make your thoughts concrete, so you can see them in black and white. So you can feel them, before they've actually happened. So you can attract that positive energy back to you. So you can take massive action!

All you really need to know is just 'the next step!' Once you take a step, then the next one becomes easier, and the next one after that, even easier than the one before! This is called flow. Once you get in the state of flow there is nothing that can stop you from achieving total wellness to honor your body, mind, soul, and spirit!

I'm pleased to bring you these healing insights to give you examples, to show you how I was able to apply them to my life. To show you how you can learn these techniques and follow the process I did. I just started with knowing the next step! I tell my oldest son that sometimes it's hard for me to explain exactly what I mean in written words. So, I hope I am making myself clear. I hope I am getting the message to you. So you can feel the hope, the healing, and the peace that I did as I discovered and took action to change my life for the better!

I hope you can feel my enthusiasm, my enlightenment, my gratitude, my sincere goodwill, and that I'm sending it out to you with this message so that you can heal just as I did. So you can design a life that nurtures every part of your being and you can have a life free of physical, emotional, and spiritual pain. Once you create a plan you will see how you draw that event back to you. Because, "When you change your energy you change your body," as Dr. Joe Dispenza describes the process. So please don't be afraid to see the possibilities. They exist! The possibilities are just waiting to be observed by you so that they can become your reality!

Healing Insight 31: You are intangible!

Tai Lopez, *67 Steps*

Tai Lopez talks about the intangibles in his *67 Steps*. Intangibles are the characteristics that we have that make us worthy of performing at our highest ability. Traits like honesty, integrity, loyalty, hard-working, strong-willed, and strong-minded. These characteristics include the will to go above and beyond. Intangibles are what lead us to excel above the average. We are all intangible! We all possess the characteristics that make us shine like no other person. It is this unique trait that helps us win the race. That helps us achieve our goals. That helps us attain superstar status. That helps us be the best that we can possibly be!

The intangibles show others what we are capable of. Think of it like this, you may not be the fastest runner on the team but because you show up every day and practice your heart out, you are the greatest asset to the team! These are the traits that make you a well-rounded person worthy of investing in. That make you worth that second chance that you were given. That make you worth the promotion you earned.

As I look back throughout my life I realize that I had more intangibles than I ever thought. I also realized that so many people along the way had seen those intangibles in me as well. But I didn't know how to process and release emotions around events and memories that were not serving me. I didn't know how to quiet my critical voice. I didn't know how to nurture my entire being. So, I didn't see many of my intangibles so clearly.

Why do we do this to ourselves? Well, it goes back to the subconscious mind running the show 95% of the day; to that 80% of our thoughts being negative and 98% of the day thinking the same thoughts that you did the day before. That's why this healing insight is included in this course. It is necessary to show you that you can shine! I want to prove to you that you have amazing abilities! You are worthy of performing to your highest ability!

I realize now that these intangibles started showing up early in my life. When I was in 3rd grade, my teacher said that I was advanced enough to push me a grade level forward. My parents said it was up to me to decide what to do. I chose to stay with my peers. Again, when I was in 6th grade, my art teacher noticed my art abilities and wanted to put me in the advanced class. I told him I would go if I could have my friend come with me. He said my friend couldn't come with me because her skills were not at that level. I refused because I didn't want to leave my friend behind. So now my art ability is limited to stick figures.

In the early 90s I was asked to relocate to Arizona to take a department manager position. I refused because of the heat. I had never been to Arizona, but I didn't even want to think about living in the heat. When I wanted to transfer (when I was two classes away from receiving my first associate degree) to pursue a second associate degree as an occupational therapist assistant, I wasn't sure if I could handle driving the 106 miles to attend class while working full-time. I mentioned my desires to one of my professors. I also expressed my doubts. She said, "You can do it!" So, I did.

When I changed jobs in March of 2012, again my intangibles shined through. Those intangibles were reflected in my pay, which ended up being that of a bachelor's degree level. When I moved to Colorado for the six months that I mentioned in Healing Insight 12, my intangibles showed up again. The owner of the Pediatric Clinic expressed her desire to have me take over the clinic when she retired, so, as you can see my intangibles showed up several times throughout my life. But I let fear make my decisions for me. By doing this, I missed opportunities. I closed doors that I should have walked through. I passed up so many chances to shine.

Sadly, in many cases, I made my choices from a state of fear which kept me from knowing that I was worthy of performing at my highest ability. But when I made the connection from this healing insight I realized that I wanted to take my life back and I was ready to heal. I'm hoping that you will take a good look at yourself. Polish those intangibles and let them shine. Use your intangibles to help you when you need to dig deep. Rely on your intangibles when you need to go above and beyond while you are on this journey!

Healing Insight 32: You need a team!

Tai Lopez, *67 Steps*

"You need a team!" Boy, Tai Lopez was right when he stressed this concept in his *67 Steps*. How true this healing insight really was. When my youngest son had difficulty getting the educational support that he needed, due to his medical conditions, I thought I could do it all. That's one of the main reasons why I went to school to get a degree in early childhood education and also for occupational therapy assistant. I felt like I had to be my son's mother, his teacher, and his therapist. I did end up attempting to fulfill all of these roles. But I'm not sure how good or bad of a job I did. I think I would rate myself on the lower end.

When my health crashed and I needed a team again, this was hard for me to accept. Yes, I got that I needed specialists for the multiple conditions that I was diagnosed with. Just as my son needed specialists for his conditions, but what I didn't get was that we could actually be a team. It would not just be providers telling me what to do with my health. I did plenty of research for all of the multiple conditions I was diagnosed with. I searched for resources to help me figure out what treatment options I had.

One resource that was especially helpful was the Interstitial Cystitis (IC) Network. They had a workbook with a flowchart of how to coordinate your health care. It also had a section for your medical team. IC Network gave support on how to realize if your medical providers were giving you adequate care. Instructions were also provided on how to go about finding and switching providers if needed. Once again, I did all the steps. I filled out all the questions. I followed through. It was a multiple-step process. I had to log in every six months to follow through with goals that I had set to improve my health, my health care, and my participation as a team player.

I realized that there were some providers that needed to be removed from my care team. I don't feel like I would have hesitated to make that decision. But this process helped me to see it so much more clearly and much sooner. When the process was all said and done, I ended up with a great team. I think maybe unknowingly, I was already quite the team player. I documented my symptoms well. Probably because I was an OT assistant and that was part of my skill set. But I questioned my treatment even more thoroughly. I tried new things. I realized that this was my team. My well-being was the focus.

I'm so glad that I understand how important a team is, especially a medical team. I'm confident and comfortable sharing my symptoms, my concerns, and my aspirations with all of my members. I'm not afraid to refuse treatment related to prescription medications. I'm not afraid to ask for alternative treatments. I know now that it is okay for me to let my medical providers know when they need to give me more support. I feel confident when I am ready to pull back or lessen that support, my medical providers will understand. That it is part of the balance that is expected and that is needed to create a medical care team to meet our individual needs.

This has been one of the most productive of my healing insights. It has helped me to realize not only that I was the focus, but I was worth it! I'm thankful for my healthcare providers as well as my ability to be a team player. I suggest that you take a look at who your team is. Remember we all need support. Just as we help so many others in our life, we need to allow others to help us as well. It is not a sign of weakness. It is a sign of wisdom to know when you need help and to be able to ask for it!

Keep in mind that the level of support you receive can always be adjusted as your health improves. Also, consider if there are any medical providers that you feel are not giving you adequate care. Adequate care includes being willing to listen to your concerns, to help you come up with a care plan that meets the needs of your mind, body, soul, and spirit. Yes, this is possible if you are willing to ask for alternative treatments! You may be surprised at the resources your medical providers may have about other ways to nurture and improve your self-care.

Healing Insight 33: Save for the rainy day.

Mela Tapia, my maternal grandmother

This healing insight was shared with me as a child, but I never applied it to my life. Sadly enough, I didn't listen to my grandmother when she would tell me, "Save for the rainy day." She was from the era of the Depression. So, she understood this well. She knew how times could change in the blink of an eye and how challenging times could linger on. She even tried to teach my children the same healing insight. She would tell them, "Put half of your money in your bank and spend half that way when you're old enough to drive you can buy yourself a car." But because I didn't reinforce this insight their savings ended up being spent before it could amount to much.

I have had financial dilemmas throughout my life and now as I have been on this journey of self-development, I realize this has been a common theme in my life. It is based on my self-worth, false beliefs, and old programs that I have around money. The biggest financial burden that I faced was when my health crashed, and I was not working. My husband was out of work again in 2015, for an entire year. I contemplated going back to work part-time. That way I could bring in some income for the rent.

Thank God for family! Between my two sons and my husband's family we were blessed to be able to survive that year. However, it was highly stressful, and it made me realize that Maslow's Hierarchy of Needs is not just a theory that I learned while working on my early childhood degree. This theory states that when your basic needs are not met, then your higher-level needs are affected. There are five levels of needs for us to feel happy and fulfilled as human beings. The five levels are, from the bottom up: physical needs like food and shelter, then safety, love, respect, and self-actualization, which are higher-level needs that include self-esteem, creativity, and problem-solving. It made a lot of sense. If you can't even have a meal, how are you going to be creative or problem solve?

Talk about being in a constant state of stress! This was one time that I should have listened to my grandmother's wisdom, but I didn't. I regretted not having anything to fall back on. Yes, I had set up a savings account in the past. But I would always end up getting into it for things that were not an emergency. So, I had nothing that I could even call savings. I felt disgusted because I chose to be foolish instead of trying to set aside some money for the rainy day that felt like a hail storm. I often wonder why

I, like many people, have chosen to learn the hard way. It makes so much more sense to learn from others so we don't have to suffer needlessly. But for some reason, this was a lesson that I was going to learn or it would defeat me.

It is difficult to stay hopeful when the chips are down. Some days I didn't know if I was coming or going. I just kept my headphones on and kept blasting new knowledge and success stories into my brain. It is the only thing I could do to keep myself from losing any ground. I had seen improvement—in my body and in my life, and I was not going to stop now. I am the optimist of the family, and I always knew that we would be blessed with the money we needed right when we needed it. I guess I was using the power of the Law of Attraction. I just had no idea what was happening. I placed my faith in a higher power and felt it in my heart that we would be taken care of.

In January of 2105, I had another pelvic surgery that included exploratory laparoscopy (lysis of adhesions, removal of endometriosis, and cyst-from my right ovary), cystoscopy, and hydrodistension (extended 30 minutes). I told myself that I was going to get back to my physical activity and yoga ASAP. I also told myself that I was not going to need pain medication. I only needed two morphine pills! I added upper body stretches and isometric exercises to maintain the strength in my muscles within the first week. I was told not to do yoga for six weeks. But I did start restorative yoga and bridges within a couple of weeks. I was feeling better in every aspect. Somehow, I believed that if I just kept applying these techniques to my life, that my body would respond in a positive way, and it did!

Even though as a society, we may not have been taught a specific name for the Law of Attraction, or we may not have been taught how the process works in school, college, or the job site, it has worked for all of us at some time or another. It is obvious that the power of positivity can make an enormous difference in your life. When you can rise above the current situation you are in, no matter how difficult, with positive thoughts you can make positive things happen in your life!

Healing Insight 34: I am not a victim!

Biology of Belief, Dr. Bruce Lipton

This is another great healing insight that gave me the knowledge and the courage to realize that I have control over my health and my life. According to Dr. Bruce Lipton, less than 1% of disease is genetic. I'm going to repeat that: *less than 1% of disease is genetic!* This was astounding to me when I first heard of it! When Dr. Lipton explained that it is what we believe that allows us to heal, he had my full attention. He went on to explain that every cell in our body has the special ability to understand our thoughts. Crazy, right? That's what I thought! I kept reading. I kept understanding how much sense it made. The power of making our thoughts matter is connected to being able to heal.

I also gained a deep respect for Dr. Lipton when he explained that he resigned from his position as a professor. He was teaching medical students. He was expected to give them false information. He was not allowed to teach the fact that our cells can heal. In the late 60s—yes the late 60s—he was doing stem cell research. What? I thought stem cell research and therapy was being viewed as cutting edge starting this past decade. He just couldn't get himself to keep this information quiet.

I also realized how powerful and selfless our cells are while reading *The Book of Secrets: Unlocking the Hidden Dimensions of Your Life* by Deepak Chopra. He explains that cells have a pro-social ability to take care of one another. They act very much like a team. I thought, wow! No wonder Bruce wrote a book, *The Wisdom of Your Cells*. I asked myself, "Where have I been and why wasn't I reading these books in my early twenties?" The bigger question is, "Why weren't these books part of our basic education?" I realized that I was not a victim even though fibromyalgia, interstitial cystitis, and irritable bowel syndrome do not have cures.

This new knowledge that only 1% of disease is genetic inspired me! Once I thought about it, I figured if genetics was not a factor then it was only related to my lifestyle. So, I just needed to clean up my lifestyle, right? It made sense! If what I was eating and what I was doing was causing me to be ill, I would change what I was doing and I could be healthy.

I remember when my rheumatologist diagnosed me with central sensitivity syndrome with fibromyalgia. My vitamin D level was severely deficient. The doctor gave me his recommendations. Vitamin D supplements were at the top of the list. He said, "Well, if you stick with the dosage of vitamin D you might feel better in more than a year, but I can't promise you." That statement both caused me fear and put a fire under my tail because I took it as a challenge. I thought to myself, how does he know I can't feel better sooner? It was a rocky road, I did have some improvements sooner, but I also had setbacks.

My old habits, programs, and false beliefs were getting the best of me. But I kept pushing forward. I kept reading books. I kept listening to these thought leaders. I consumed their knowledge. Their stories empowered me! Their challenges inspired me! I thought, wow, so many of these individuals have overcome feats much greater than mine. Surely, I should be able to improve my lifestyle and improve my health. Gaining this knowledge helped me to take massive action! Listening to the success stories along with this new knowledge helped me quiet my critical voice. I knew that I needed a whole new mindset. I did need to reprogram my mind like many of these thought leaders recommended.

So that's how I used the many books, self-development courses, webinars, videos, and emails. I chose to create a new mindset, to reprogram my mind, to take a leap of faith and believe in myself. I put my intangibles to work for me, and I started making decisions based on love. I chose to love and honor my mind, body, soul, and spirit! This journey has been challenging. Yes, the steps are simple. Thanks to all the knowledge of how the brain and body work the steps become effortless! I am so grateful for all the wonderful thought leaders that are not afraid to share their knowledge, to share the hope, and to lend a helping hand. I just kept thinking, they don't even know me and look how much they've helped me. Now that's love!

Healing Insight 35: We are interdependent.

The 7 Habits of Highly Effective People, Stephen R. Covey

This was probably one of the toughest healing insights for me to believe. This healing insight was one of the main concepts I learned from the book, *The 7 Habits of Highly Effective People* by Stephen R. Covey. As I mentioned, in Healing Insight 15 I moved out when I was 16 years old, and I have been independent ever since, or so I thought. I was always so proud of being an independent woman, a working woman, an educated woman, a strong woman, a woman who didn't need anyone for anything.

I think that's why I was so hard on myself and others. I had the misconception that you had to do it on your own, that you only had yourself. Even though I had great support from my father, my grandmother, my husband, my boys, some very close aunts, uncles, cousins, and friends, I still felt as though I couldn't ask for anyone's help. I couldn't show anyone that I was weak. I couldn't express any fear. I thought I had to always maintain the persona of a tough, independent woman.

Had I realized this insight earlier in my life and accepted it as a reasonable, intelligent, life-preserving concept, maybe I could have asked for some help when I knew I was totally overwhelmed. Instead, I just kept pushing, pushing, pushing. I kept ignoring my body, ignoring my symptoms, ignoring my pain, ignoring my emotions, until my body fell apart. I had pain from head to toe. I was miserable. I was weak. But I was still trying to convince myself that I could do it all alone.

After my surgery in 2012, the doctor gave me a lifetime restriction. I was told that I could never lift anything over 35 pounds. In 2014, after the car accident, my physical therapist restricted me from lifting my arms above my head, with or without weights. That meant if I needed to reach for something on a shelf above my head I couldn't do it myself. I was frustrated and angry because I hated that I now had to ask for help and I couldn't do things I was used to doing for myself and by myself. I felt worthless because I viewed myself as sooo damn independent. I felt insulted that I needed anyone's help.

"We are stronger together than we are alone."

~Walter Payton~

This quote is magical to me because it shows how needing other people, being interdependent, is not a weakness but a sign of strength. It shows unity. It shows a connection. It shows how being interdependent is a wise choice. I truly do appreciate this healing insight. It has taught me to be able to appreciate my family more. It has helped me to understand how much they really do for me. How much they really care for me. And how much they really love me. It has shown me how great we are when we work together. How strong we are when we support one another. How unified we are when we rely on one another.

However, my pride proved to be a deeper issue than I thought. I kept feeling frustrated and angry. Then I felt guilty. I felt like I was a burden to my family. I felt like every time I asked them for help I was bothering them.

I finally decided to be clear with my family and tell them ahead of time what I needed help with. I asked them to try to help me with those tasks even if I did not ask them to. This helped a great deal. I did have to remind them or ask them if they forgot but for the most part, it made me realize that this situation was not as bad as I was making it.

The point I'm trying to make is that I was focusing on the negative, again. Honestly, I was feeling sorry for myself, too. As an OT assistant, I had been taught how difficult role changes are during illness and loss of function. But I didn't realize how emotional it would be. I couldn't see how blessed I was. I couldn't see how valuable each of us was to this family unit. I couldn't see the value that I still had. Tapping Meditation helped me to give all of these emotions a voice. This technique helped me to finally process and release emotions not serving me. So just remember it's okay to be interdependent; this is the best way to honor your mind, body, soul, and spirit.

Healing Insight 36: You can have heaven on Earth!

How to Live Heaven on Earth (YouTube), Dr. Bruce Lipton

Because we are the creators of our own reality, we can have heaven on Earth. When I first heard this healing insight I had my doubts. I thought, I have wanted heaven on Earth and I have not achieved it. So how can this be true? It's simple. I didn't have the knowledge that I could even be happy internally.

I was always relying on my external reality for my happiness. Sure, I was a happy person in general. I was optimistic. But I was totally dependent on the moods, actions, and reactions of other people to determine my own happiness. I was always trying to please others, to make others happy so that I could be happy. That didn't work because they obviously didn't have a clue either. So, there was a whole lot of unhappiness going around.

Understanding how to be happy now rather than seeking happiness was a concept that was hard to wrap my mind around. I always believed happiness was the end result of accomplishments, material items, and money. We are taught that once we win the race we will be happy. Rather than basking in the happiness of being in the race, we are taught that we can't be happy until we get that something that we desire. Instead, we need to realize that happiness is the process, not the product.

I had it all wrong. No wonder I always seemed puzzled and downright frustrated. When I finally achieved what was supposed to make me happy I realized I was not happy. I thought, wait a minute, what did I miss? I did everything I was supposed to do. I created a goal. I worked hard. I accomplished the goal. So, where in the hell is the happiness? I felt cheated. I felt stupid. I felt disappointed. I felt disgusted. I felt defeated.

We must start with happiness, with gratitude, with appreciation, and with a sense of peace. The rest will fall into place. It sounds so simple, and it is once you know the formula. You can have heaven on earth. You must discover that the hope, the healing, and the peace are all part of happiness. You must figure out that, "Heaven is a state and not a place," Anita Moorjani.

Once you accept this healing insight as a new belief you don't have to rush. You don't have to worry. You don't have to beat the clock to get where you're going. You can wake up and already be happy. Then you can create the life you deserve. I know this is a completely different mindset. But please take the time to learn it. It will make all the difference in your life.

This healing insight will allow you to enjoy every moment of your waking hours. It will allow you to be more present. It will allow you to look forward to the day. It will allow you to realize how precious your time is. It will allow you to realize how precious you are. It will allow you to realize how precious your loved ones are. It will allow you to enjoy that time together. It will allow you to create memories and experiences that are truly free of worry and stress. It will help you to realize what really matters to you. It will allow you to surround yourself with what really brings you joy!

Healing Insight 37: The secret to living is giving.

MONEY Master the Game, Tony Robbins

Lack is a survival emotion. It is one of many in this category which includes insecurity, hatred, judgment, victimization, worry, guilt, depression, shame, anxiety, regret, suffering, frustration, fear, greed, sadness, disgust, envy, anger, resentment, and unworthiness. Dr. Joe Dispenza talks about how detrimental these survival emotions are in his book, *Breaking the Habit of Being Yourself.* This is very important to know when you're trying to heal! If you stay stuck in these survival emotions, even in just one of them, you start feeling the others more and more because they are a package deal. Before you know it, you are stuck in the stress response cycle which causes you to be in a state of scarcity.

What does giving have to do with survival emotions, especially lack? Giving helps you automatically get out of the state of scarcity. It helps reframe your mindset. It helps you feel abundant. Robert Kiyosaki explains this in his book, *Rich Dad Poor Dad.* His biological father was a very giving man. But because he was in the mindset of scarcity, he thought he had to pay the bills first then if there was something left he would give to charity. This mindset kept him from regularly donating to charity and kept him feeling the survival emotion of lack. On the other hand, his Rich Dad, the gentleman from whom he learned financial wisdom, would take his pay from his business earnings and donate to charity first. This allowed him to access the state of an abundant mindset.

When I was growing up, I was taught to give to charity. Or to those that were less fortunate. I remember numerous times when we would stop and give money to those standing on the side of the road. We would donate clothing and household items to our local charities. We would donate non-perishable items to the local food drive events. But this concept of giving before paying your bills and making it a consistent habit every month was just amazing to me! Tony Robbins suggests that you have three spending jars. One marked as ours, one marked as friends & family to help friends and family members, and one marked people you don't know to donate to. I thought, wow, I can't even have one savings account much less three!

The mindset of abundance allows this to happen. You don't have to start big. You can decide like I did to give $5 to a different charity every month. If your local community is having back-to-school supply drives or food drives in the grocery stores just make a promise to yourself that each time you go to the grocery store you will donate $1 to that cause. If you can't donate every single time you go in, please understand that at least you need to donate one time. This small act of kindness will set you free from the survival emotion of lack. It will help you get out of this stress response cycle. It will help you realize how good you can feel by knowing that your state of welfare is better than it seems because you believe that way.

Think of this quote: "What is Faith? When we accept a thought independent of the conditions in our environment and then surrender to the outcome to such a degree that we live as if our prayers are already answered," Dr. Joe Dispenza.

If finances are truly not available to you, don't feel bad. Don't feel guilty. There are other ways to provide a donation. Remember you can give some household items that you're not using anymore. Or you can even donate one or two cans of non-perishable items to the local food bank. Also, your time is a wonderful gift. Maybe you could read to your child's classroom. Or maybe donate some books that you are not using to the local library. There are so many ways to give. Giving some time to listen to someone in need is a great gift altogether. It's a wonderful way to help you take your focus off of yourself, your pain, and your burdens.

Tony Robbins revealed that research showed how happiness is directly related to how people used their money. Their happiness was increased when they gave money to someone they didn't know. It allowed them to feel those higher-level emotions of service, joy, peace, love, freedom, inspiration, and abundance. So, give it a try! Once you can feel those higher-level emotions, you are accessing the part of your being that helps you heal. Plus, you will be in a much more positive state of mind!

This healing insight is an amazing mindset shift! I hope you can implement this new belief today. Remember the amount does not matter. It could even be pennies that you save in a bank for the whole month. Then donate them when you go into the local grocery store that has a can for donations for any cause. The effect is the same. It will shift your mindset to a state of abundant thinking. It will make you feel better. The benefits are great and felt by your entire being: your body, mind, soul, and spirit! So, create a space to heal by realizing that the secret to living is giving!

Healing Insight 38: What is the one thing I can do such that by doing it everything else will be easier or unnecessary?

The ONE Thing: The Surprisingly Simple Truth Behind Extraordinary People, Gary W. Keller and Jay Papasan

This healing insight taught me about focus, about possibility, and about ability. When you focus on one thing, then all of your energy is placed on that one thing. Think about it. By focusing on this one thing it also helps you prioritize and recognize what you should be focusing on. I realized that my mind was in too many places at once. I was not accomplishing anything. I was worried, angry, frustrated, and reactive. Obviously, I wasn't focused on healing. I was focused on all of the negative aspects that had gotten me exactly where I was at that point in my life. I was still thinking the same thoughts, having the same feelings, the same emotions, and doing the same things that have gotten me sick.

I started noticing that there was a common theme in all of the books I was reading. Every successful person had a system in place to nurture their mind, body, soul, and spirit. How simple. I thought, how stupid of me. I was actually dumbfounded. I thought, damn, I can't get the right programs—is it too late for me? I realized that I needed to reset my mind and re-organize my life. This book confirmed the best way to structure your life for success was to take care of yourself.

In summary, this was what I learned. You get up. You do some type of meditation, whether it's praying, 'Tapping,' or traditional meditation. You exercise, you shower, you have a meal with your family, and then you're ready to work. Now you focus the first four hours of your work day to get the most important things done. You focus on 'the one thing' that needs to get done at that moment. You do the most important thing first. You don't wait until the end of the day to do it.

I also learned from the book *The Story of the Human Body* by Daniel Lieberman that we only have a certain amount of glycogen (sugar bursts) per day. Essentially that equates to energy. So, if you think about it, we usually have the most energy, and we are the freshest at the first part of the day. That means we should be doing those activities that are the most important to us so we can focus on the most important thing. We can use the most energy and get the most benefit early in the day.

So, you should be doing the most important thing at the start of your day, which is taking care of yourself. You should clear your mind of negative thoughts. Spend some time in that inner peace with sprit because meditation is the second-best way to heal your body besides sleep. You should get some movement because movement is organizing to the brain and helps decrease anxiety, depression, and stress. You should then nourish your body with a healthy meal. Then spend some time with your family to have that connection. Build those relationships, nurture them, and then run off to work to do the best that you can do for that day.

If you're not working outside the home, then you're thinking this doesn't apply to me. BS, it applies to you even more! Implement this into your life and then focus on what is 'the one thing' that you should be doing that day. Ask yourself, "What is 'the one thing' I should be focusing on? Is it releasing anger? Is it quieting that critical voice? Is it helping to relieve stress? By going for a walk or getting some type of movement? Is it revamping my idea of what a healthy meal is by doing a little bit of research?"

This is a vital piece to creating a space to heal! These steps set your central nervous system up to be able to be balanced, so you can access the parasympathetic nervous system which is responsible for healing your body. I know this is difficult. I was not taught to take care of myself in this way. But it is mandatory if you expect to take back your health, get control of your life, and find relief today!

Whatever that looks like for you, whatever your level is right now, is fine. You don't have to meditate or exercise for an hour. You can do a 1-minute meditation and a 5-minute yoga routine. These may sound like little steps that won't get you anywhere. But with consistent repetition, your body will be primed for healing. You will start making those changes to heal your mind, your body, your soul, and your spirit! So, take action today!

Healing Insight 39: War Room Journal

War Room Prayer is a Powerful Weapon, the creators of *Fireproof* and *Courageous*

This healing insight has been so healing, fulfilling, and uplifting to me. Have you ever watched *The War Room* movie? It's based on different individuals and their perception of the hustle and bustle of their daily lives. It explains how easily we get caught up in all the stuff that is not important. It emphasizes how we lose sight of what we should truly be grateful for. Best of all it shows you how to focus on gratitude and the important things in your life. It gives you an outlet for how to deal with struggle, challenge, and arguments.

The 'war room journal' that I created while implementing this healing insight into my own daily life has become a precious treasure to me. Not only did I add scriptures to my 'war room journal,' but I also wrote personal prayers to help me find the hope, the healing, and the peace in my own personal life. I also added my favorite quotes, mantras, and my favorite personal development activities. I took it a step further, by using the 'war room journal' daily. I not only wrote uplifting scriptures but also recited the prayers with my husband each morning to help us set the tone for the day.

The basic concept of the 'war room' is to list all your challenges and emotions on a piece of paper. Clear the walls and de-clutter the room. That way you have zero distractions. Now you can focus on those items that need your attention. Then you go to war with whatever challenges you have. You write your scriptures, and you say your prayers, surrounding the challenges that you are battling.

The process is supposed to help you realize that you're waging war on the wrong thing when you are battling with the loved ones in your life. It shows you how to turn to faith and face those challenges in a more uplifting, peaceful way. I know the power of prayer and its importance throughout my life, so I did the 'war room' process. Then I transferred my scriptures. My personal prayers. My thoughts. My deepest emotions and challenges to my 'war room journal.'

I am not trying to guide you toward any religion. That is not the point here. The point is to lead you to spirituality. To help you find a more humane approach to the daily challenges that we face. To help you realize that if you focus on gratitude, you can find a solution. You can find a way to remove the craziness from your heart, your mind, your body, and your home.

The funny thing is when we went to watch this movie, we thought it was some type of an actual war movie. I learned so much from this movie, and from this process. I am grateful that we misunderstood the title and went to watch it. This is a whole new way of dealing with challenges. A whole new mindset! It is a whole new way to journal. So, give it a try. Allow yourself to open up, to create a space to heal by realizing how much you have to be grateful for. Understand that the real challenges do not lie with the people that you share your life with, but with the emotions tied to these challenges. Remember, action is what makes changes happen. In your body, and in your life!

Please do not take these healing insights lightly. They have healed me inside and out! Try these activities for yourself. As they work for you, turn them into daily habits and create your new healthy lifestyle!

Healing Insight 40: Frustration is a product of our expectations.

The 7 Habits of Highly Effective People, Stephen R. Covey

This is another great healing insight from *The 7 Habits of Highly Effective People.* This insight clearly defines how and why our frustrations are related to our expectations. I believe the expectations that we place on ourselves as well as those that society places on us can lead to great heights of frustration. This book taught me that expectations being placed on us by society do not necessarily match our values or beliefs. Many times, the expectations that are placed on us are inappropriate, unfair, and are just downright ridiculous.

Because we are so critical, we tend to place unreasonable expectations on ourselves, so these expectations are not always achievable, or they do not always take our emotional well-being into consideration. Expectations that are placed on us by family, friends, co-workers, employers, and society can cause huge frustration since we have little to no control of them. So how can we deal with this frustration and expectations that hinder us instead of supporting us?

First, you must recognize whose expectations they are. If they are your own expectations, then you need to listen to that critical voice. See what needs to be worked on. Process and release those emotions so that you can see the good in the situation. So that appropriate expectations can be made and met. If these expectations are placed on us by others or society, you must determine if you want to be held accountable for them or not. I know it is not always easy and it doesn't seem like you have a choice, but you do.

You can learn techniques of time management, stress relief, and self-coping skills. Also, you can learn how to say no—even to the most important people in your life. These techniques will help you not to fill your plate with expectations that are meaningless. Once time management, stress relief, and coping skills are in place, they will help you to meet expectations that are attainable. This will help reduce procrastination and relieve tension around not having enough time. It will also improve productivity so that expectations can be met in a reasonable timeframe.

Again, mindset is a factor related to this healing insight. It is not so much what the expectation is but how you perceive it. Even just changing from a scarcity to an abundant mindset can help you realize if expectations are reasonable. This will help you decide if you should be responsible for them. If expectations do not have your best interest at heart, then you need to evaluate how you can use other skills to minimize the amount of expectations that are placed on you. Even the simplest ways of excusing yourself from a task or an expectation that was asked of you can relieve so much frustration. This will allow you to honor your mind, body, soul, and spirit by giving you a voice in what tasks and expectations you are responsible for.

Some ways that you can accomplish this is by simply saying; "I would love to help you but I'm feeling like I'm not the right person for this." Then provide a resource. Or you can say, "Right now, I'm focusing on my personal well-being. I have committed six weeks to myself. So, I am not taking on any other tasks." Believe me the ability to say no is the best skill you can acquire in your life. It will keep you from being pressured into things that you feel are not necessary, not your responsibility and many times just a waste of your time and energy. It is a skill that needs to be honed. The sooner you start using it, the better you will be at being diplomatic, polite, and sincere when declining.

Remember, this book is to teach you how to create a space to heal. To start nurturing your entire being. To be able to apply self-care to all levels of your life. You must remember you matter! Your time matters. Your energy matters. Your mind, your body, your soul, and your spirit matter! Take these steps to heal yourself so you can create the life you deserve! So you can live a full life!

Healing Insight 41: Thoughts matter!

All Thought Leaders

This healing insight will allow you to realize to what degree your thoughts matter. Dr. Joe Dispenza took my understanding of the Law of Attraction to a deeper, higher, more spiritual level. In his book, *You Are the Placebo: Making Your Mind Matter,* he explains this concept. He helped me connect so many loose ends and so many questions; he helped me understand how you must not just think a thought; you must feel it, in every fiber of your being. You must observe that desire as if it has already taken place. You must send out that positive energy and surrender your mind, body, soul, and spirit completely! Then and only then are you capable of attracting all that your heart desires!

This healing insight helps you realize how you can transcend your body, time, your environment, and space. It helps you realize that time is not linear. Time does not happen in the straight sequence of past, present, or future. It will help you understand what to focus on. Dr. Dispenza explains, "Wherever you place your attention is where you place your energy." It will help you understand that you need access to the full amount of your energy to be able to make a positive impact in your life. I didn't totally understand the concept of needing your full energy until I took James Van Praagh's free online course, *One Day to Unconditional Self-Love.*

Mr. Van Praagh helped me realize that when you are placing your focus (your energy) on judging others, trying to change others, trying to help others, and trying to make others happy, you are not focusing on yourself. Your energy is tied up with that other person. So, you don't have access to the full amount of your energy. He also explained that you are taking away and consuming the other person's energy. So, if you really want to help someone, you must release that judgment, release that need to control, and release that need to help them. Remember, each of us has everything we need inside of us to be successful. But to achieve that success, we need to access the full amount of our energy. Now I completely understand what Mr. Van Praagh meant about needing to clear your energy and protect it daily.

This healing insight also helped me realize how successful individuals make their thoughts matter. They mentally rehearse their physical actions over and over and over until it is perfected in their mind and they feel it in their soul so that they can take action to make it become a reality. This technique works for athletes, actors, and singers. Dr. Bruce Lipton said, "Repetition is one of the four ways that programs can be changed." Repetition is useful when you are building a new healthy habit. But it is detrimental when you have a habit that's not serving you, because it is the repetition that makes the habit so strong and subconscious in your mind.

You must understand this healing insight, because it is at the core of the healing process, the core of detox, the core of releasing emotion, the core of mindset, the core of reprogramming your mind, and the core of exercise/physical activity. It is the foundation of The 5-Step Process that I have created in the 70-Day Course.

I encourage you to read all of Dr. Joe Dispenza's books. Embrace his knowledge. Apply it to your life. Once you do, you will see miraculous changes! In your mind, in your body, in your soul, and in your spirit, as well as in your life! Your reality will become something that you can build just by thought!

The secret to this process is basking in the emotions of gratitude ahead of time. Yes, be grateful for future blessings. Feel all those emotions that you usually do when you have received a blessing. This will help you experience the higher-level emotions, so you can feel that thought. When you send out that positive energy, your thoughts and your feelings will match, which sends out a positive invitation to the universe. Once you surrender completely, you will attract what you send out, and your thoughts will become a reality!

This healing insight will help you cement in your mind how a positive outlook, positive thoughts, and positive mindset must be practiced daily. Gratitude is the force behind using the Law of Attraction to the fullest benefit of your well-being. So that you can maximize for a full life; so that you can live a pain-free life and love every minute of it! We may not have been taught this healing insight as children. Maybe we didn't realize our life's purpose early in our lives. That's okay. We can apply this healing insight by using the Law of Attraction to develop our mind, body, soul, and spirit completely and consistently. So we can live a truly enlightened life!

Activity:

"Positively Grateful!"

Instructions:

- List 5 positively great things someone has done for you.

- List 5 positively great things you have done for others.

- Be "Positively Grateful" for all the acts of kindness you have been blessed to give and receive!

"Positively Grateful!" Activity Sheet

Great Things You Have Received	Great Things You Have Given

Daily Challenge:

Turn Hope into Action!

"Create Your Reality!"

"Create Your Reality" with one of these amazing thoughts today!

- "I Feel Amazing!"

- "I Am Wonderful!"

- "I Am Positive!"

- "I Am Safe!"

- "I Am Enough!"

Remember: You can't just think an amazing thought!

- You must feel it, in every fiber of your being!

- You must observe this amazing thought as if it has already taken place!

- You must send out that positive energy and surrender your mind, body, soul, and spirit completely!

- Now attract all that your heart desires!

Healing Insight 42: Know your leading energy.

Tony Robbins, Email Newsletter

This healing insight shocked me because my entire life I thought that I was masculine energy. But what I learned helped me realize why I have been acting this way for all these years. This was another benefit of signing up for email newsletters that proved to be super valuable! There was a quiz in the email I received from Tony Robbins, to determine your leading energy.

Once again, I convinced my husband that we should take the quiz. We did his quiz first. I read the questions to him as he mostly answered. I would answer ahead of him at times. When he was uncertain, I would kind of guide him to answer what I thought was correct. He jokingly said, "You don't know me." We went through the same questions to get the results of my quiz. We were both shocked with what our leading energy is!

My husband's leading energy is masculine, and my leading energy is feminine. I always thought that his energy was feminine and, as I said, mine masculine. I was puzzled, I wondered, did we answer the questions right? It just didn't seem right with the way that our personalities are. The way we interact with each other. I've always been bold and blunt and tough. My husband is extremely verbal, and he will stand up for himself initially, but he withdraws, and he will shut down and back off. This is why it was such a shock once we were given the results.

An explanation came with the results. It explained that masculine leading energy would demonstrate feminine leading energy characteristics as a defense mechanism. The same was true for the feminine energy. It would take on masculine energy traits when that person felt threatened or thought they needed to be defensive. This was happening because my husband and I had not been communicating to one another correctly. We had not been speaking the correct love language to each other because we didn't have a clue.

This explained why we were causing one another to go into defense mode when we were so upset with one another. It just became a habit. It is what we did during all the stressful situations in our lives. The fact that we did not have a coping skill to process and release the emotions that were holding us back and not serving us, is what caused us to be in constant stress response cycle. That is why we appeared to be the opposite leading energy.

I believe that I have been exhibiting this masculine energy my entire life because I have been defending myself or thinking that I needed to defend myself. I have been using the masculine energy traits as a guard with strained relationships, especially the one with my mother. Then this masculine energy just continued through my marriage and throughout my life.

The fact that my husband and I were raised with a scarcity mindset didn't help matters. Because we came from that type of background, we didn't know anything different. So, we had been experiencing and feeling all the survival emotions. The emotions had kept us in that stress response cycle. This led us to show signs of the opposite leading energy.

I reread the explanation several times. Every time I read it, the facts became more real to me. It confirmed that my scarcity mindset, my sense of lack, and being in chronic stress response cycle pretty much my entire life had placed me in the defensive state. I didn't know myself. So, I guess my husband was right, I didn't know him. How could I? I didn't even know myself! Wow! Again, I felt like this is information that should have been taught to me in school was never there. How necessary it is to know this. To know when you're stuck in the chronic stress response cycle.

It's no wonder my health crashed! It's a miracle that it lasted as long as it did! I don't know if I should be mad or sad when I think of this. I have so many mixed emotions, but I was relieved that at least now I knew what my leading energy was. I was thankful that I understood why I was displaying features of the opposite leading energy. I was grateful to have this new knowledge. I am blessed to be able to continue to use the Tapping Meditation Process to help me release emotions not serving me. As they show up in my life, this will allow me to be my leading energy. So I can be that soft feminine energy that I lost years ago. Or maybe I never truly even had the chance to develop my leading energy.

I recommend that you sign up for Tony Robbins' email newsletters. Better yet, take the leading energy quiz! You owe it to yourself! Find out what your leading energy is so you can find your true self! Discover who you really are! Be your true self! You are amazing! But you may not even know it. You may not even know who you are. Connect with your true self so that you can find the state of balance that you deserve! So you can create a space to heal and you can live your full life!

Healing Points to Treasure

1. The Law of Attraction, "like attracts like," has the power to make you the creator of your destiny. Use it to the benefit of your own well-being. Teach your children and your grandchildren how to maximize for a full life!

2. Make your decisions from love, not fear. Fear keeps you from knowing the next step because it is a survival emotion. Remember when you start experiencing one survival emotion, it's a package deal.

3. Intangibles are the characteristics that make you worthy of performing at your highest ability. You possess the characteristics that make you shine like no other person.

4. Understand how important a team is. Remember you need support. Just as you help so many others in your life, you need to allow others to help you as well.

5. Financial dilemmas are based on self-worth, false beliefs, and old programs you have around money. Use the power of positivity to rise above the current situation, no matter how difficult. You can make positive things happen in your life with positive thoughts!

6. If only 1% of disease is genetic, then genetics is not a huge factor, as once believed. Illness is related to lifestyle. So, you just need to clean up your lifestyle!

7. Realize how valuable the family unit is. Being interdependent is not a weakness, it is a sign of strength. It is a misconception that you must do it on your own, that you only have yourself.

8. Because you are the creator of your own reality, you can have heaven on Earth. This healing insight will allow you to enjoy every moment of your waking hours. Realize that happiness is the process, not the product.

9. Giving helps you automatically get out of the state of scarcity. It helps reframe your mindset. It helps you feel abundant!

10. When you focus on one thing, all your energy is placed on that one thing! This will teach you focus, possibility, and how to access your ability. You should be doing the most important thing, which is taking care of yourself at the start of the day.

11. The journaling process shows you how to focus on gratitude and the important things in your life. It gives you an outlet for how to deal with struggle, challenge, and arguments.

12. Mindset is a factor related to frustration around expectations. It is not so much what the expectation is but how you perceive it. Changing from a scarcity to an abundant mindset can help you realize if expectations are reasonable.

13. Realize to what degree your thoughts matter. This healing insight is the foundation of The 5-Step Process that I have created. Your reality will become something that you can build just by thought!

14. Discover who you really are! You are amazing! But you may not even know it. You may not even know who you are.

CHAPTER FOUR

Step 4 Reprogramming Your Mind: Healing Insights 43–56

The secret to this process is basking in the emotions of gratitude ahead of time. Feel all those emotions that you usually do when you have received a blessing. Once you surrender completely you will attract what you send out. Your thoughts will become a reality!

I wasn't doing myself any favors thinking negative thoughts and being in a constant state of anger. This vicious cycle stopped me from finding the hope, the healing, and the peace. I didn't know how to access the healing power of my subconscious mind. I had so many negative thoughts I was swimming in a pool of pain, grief, and despair. I had to learn that I was the placebo!

What I was about to learn about reprogramming my mind would change me from the inside out! What I share with you will help you realize to what degree you must change. How your conscious and subconscious mind works as a team. How positive thoughts and feelings are the ingredients to access the healing power of your subconscious mind. I will show you how I was able to heal my mind, body, soul, and spirit!

In this chapter you will learn the process of acceptance to become your own friend. This alone is a huge factor in your ability to reprogram your mind. You will finally understand how to access the healing power of your subconscious mind! You will learn how to send out abundance invitations. You will realize how gratitude is the only way to maintain a positive mindset to attract abundance. You will learn how to improve relationships and heal yourself! You will be given the steps to create your reality by thought alone!

Healing Insight 43: Be your own friend, forgive, love, and nurture yourself.

Jessica Ortner, The Tapping Solution

This healing insight has helped me realize how to create a sanctuary for my mind, body, soul, and spirit. I didn't believe I was worthy of love and I neglected my needs. Also, forgiveness was a great struggle for me. But this healing insight gave me permission to forgive, love, and nurture myself without holding back. It is so dear to my heart because it helped me to nurture my inner child. It helped me heal lifelong wounds. It helped me process and release sadness, sorrow, and grief that was not serving me or anyone else. It helped me value my emotions, give them a voice, and let them go. So I could heal every fiber of my being.

This healing insight gave me the fundamental building blocks to implement self-care for every part of my being. It showed me that I am not my thoughts. It taught me how not only to listen to my mind and critical voice but to know what I need to 'Tap on.' It taught me to listen to my pain. To know what my body needed. It taught me to listen to my soul. To know what emotions needed to be processed and released. It helped me to listen to my spirit; to live my truth, my purpose, and realize my full potential.

Jessica Ortner explains how you must be your own friend. Think about it. What things does your critical voice tell you every day? If you would tell your friends and family the things you tell yourself, you wouldn't have anyone around you. I know I would be all alone if I would have said these things to anyone but myself. So why do you think it's okay to talk to yourself that way? Why do you think it's okay to mistreat yourself? Why do you think it's okay to torture yourself?

The reason is simple. We haven't nurtured our mind, body, soul, and spirit. We have barely met the basic needs of our body like food and shelter.

Maslow's Hierarchy of Needs

Essentially, we are only surviving and not living. We have not even done a good job of meeting the mid or higher-level needs listed on Maslow's Hierarchy of Needs pyramid. This simple psychology theory plainly states that if your basic needs are not met, you cannot reach the higher levels. I mentioned this in Healing Insight 33 but let's discuss its importance further. How is Maslow's Hierarchy of Needs related to this healing insight? If you don't nurture yourself and if all your needs are not met, you cannot realize your full potential. If you cannot realize your full potential, you cannot achieve it. In fact, even if you just think or perceive that you don't have the resources to meet your basic needs you will remain stuck in the stress response cycle.

Think of it like this, when you are threatened or even feel that you are threatened your body goes into the stress response mode. Because you don't have coping skills to process and release those emotions that are not serving you, you stay stuck in the stress response cycle. You continue to believe that your basic needs are not being met. You don't feel safe or secure. So, you can't focus on your psychological needs which include love and relationships. Now you don't even feel loved so how can you have good self-esteem? You can't! So, you keep thinking and feeling like none of your needs are being met. Your thoughts make your body keep you in a chronic stress response cycle. You are still thinking your needs are not being met. So, you will never reach the highest level which is self-fulfillment needs. You will never feel or be fulfilled. You will never see your full potential. You will never reach your full potential! Also, lack of self-care has robbed you of creating a life you deserve. It has made you believe that you don't matter. That you are not worthy of friendship, forgiveness, and love, not even from yourself.

It saddens me to point this out. But I am honored that I can help you create a space to heal. I'm so thankful that I can share these healing insights with you. I feel empowered knowing that the techniques I teach you will change your life forever! I am blessed to offer you this wisdom so you can live a pain-free life and love every minute of it! I hope that you can understand how vital this healing insight is for your healing, your enjoyment of life, and to achieve your full potential! Let this healing insight work its amazing healing wonders in your body and in your life. Feel the calm and the safety that it showers you with. Indulge in its power to heal your mind, body, soul, and spirit!

Healing Insight 44: You are only responsible for your own happiness.

The Tapping World Summit 2015

Wow! This healing insight was absolute freedom for me! I had been trying to make too many people happy my entire life, including myself. This concept was one of the greatest that I could have ever learned from The Tapping World Summit 2015. It was so powerful because I had also just learned that happiness is within. So, the day I learned about this healing insight, I was overwhelmed with emotion. I think I felt every emotion that I could have felt in that moment. I experienced joy, anger, frustration, acceptance, and love.

I 'Tapped and Tapped' again to calm myself. To help myself process everything that I had just heard and every emotion I had. Tears were streaming down my face. Finally, I was free! I didn't have to try to make people happy because it didn't work anyway. I realized, at that moment, that I didn't even know how to be happy. So how did I expect to make other people happy? I had been stuffing down emotions, holding back, limiting myself, walking on eggshells, holding my tongue, trying not to rock the boat, trying to be the glue, trying to be the peacemaker, and trying to keep balance my entire life.

Now the floodgates were open. I didn't know how to handle this. I felt like I needed to totally release my burden of trying to make my husband happy all these years. I was going to wait until the right time to break this news to him, so I thought. But when I walked into the bedroom, I knew I had to speak to him at that moment. He was still in bed resting. It was a Saturday, I believe. I said, "I need to talk to you. I have something to tell you." I knelt on the side of the bed, opposite of him. I started 'Tapping' on my chest because immediately I was anxious and fearful of what I might say and how it would be perceived by my husband.

I just declared, "I am not responsible for your happiness. As a matter of fact, I'm not responsible for trying to make anybody happy. Only myself. All these years, I've been carrying this burden, and I have been trying to make you happy. I've been trying to make my mom happy, and I've been trying to make myself happy. I don't even know how to do that for myself. I've been so foolish to think that I could make anyone else happy. I can't do this anymore. It's killing me inside. It's too heavy for me to carry. Now I know that I don't have to. So as of today, I will no longer try to make you happy because that is on you. This is not on my plate. I'm putting it in your ball court. You can be sad, happy, or whatever you end up being. But it's not my fault because I am not responsible for your happiness. Just like I am not responsible for trying to make my mother happy. I don't even need you or my mother to make me happy. Because now I know that happiness is within." I cried and 'Tapped.'

Eventually, I got myself together, and I told him, "I love you, but your happiness is your responsibility or your burden, however you want or choose to look at it. But it is not mine." I think he was in shock. I'm not even sure if it was disbelief or if he was still just in a state of sleepiness that I caught him in, so off-guard. He really didn't respond. Or maybe he was still processing all the information and all the emotion that had just been dumped on him.

I was free. I was cleansed. I felt amazing! I was happy, probably for the first time in my entire life. Because I knew that I had control of my life and only my life. I didn't have to be burdened with anyone else or their emotions. Amen! This was so uplifting that I'm cheerful and emotional as I share this healing insight with you! I don't know what you've been taught. I don't know what your beliefs are around happiness or being responsible for anyone else's happiness. Whatever your beliefs are, I want to help you understand this healing insight because this is at the center of your emotional well-being. This is what I keep referring to. That you must not only take care of your mind and your body but also your soul and your spirit. This is the beginning of your healing!

I hope you will not view this healing insight as silly or overemphasized. This healing insight will not only heal your entire being, it will help you nurture your emotional well-being! It will help you connect with your soul, to your true self, to spirit. Allow this insight to settle into your mind, body, soul, and spirit! Feel it at every level so you can find the hope, the healing, and the peace!

Healing Insight 45: Your mind is unilateral; stop multitasking!

All Thought Leaders

This healing insight has been quite difficult for me to comprehend as well as apply to my life. It is not that I can't understand that our mind can only do one thing at a time. It's that I have been multitasking for so long, it's all I know. I often would tell my oldest son, other family members, and even friends that I thought I might have attention deficit disorder. When I was multitasking, I felt as if I couldn't focus on just one thing. I felt like I was bobbing back and forth from everything. If you think about it that is exactly what I was doing, no wonder I felt like I had ADD.

But the simple fact is, our conscious mind can only focus on one thing. We cannot multitask. We can only switch attention from one activity to the other. But there is a lag time of a few seconds before we can focus again on the other task, this causes us to lose or miss information. If we are multitasking the reality is that we don't end up getting anything accomplished because we are switching back and forth between many tasks and not achieving what we set out to do.

All the thought leaders recognize this to be true. Dr. Hyman, as well as Tony Robbins, have specific articles about this topic that is sent out to their followers in email format. Tony Robbins has emphasized that women tend to be more prone to multitasking since we have many responsibilities which include looking after our families. This is thought to be the main reason why men are more successful because they can focus on one thing.

Another reason why I think so many of us are prone to multitasking is because we are not present. We do not live in the here and now. We are constantly in the past, in the future, trying to figure out what we need to do next. How we need to prepare or what we need to plan. For that reason, we are don't feel like we can spend time focusing on one thing. Because we are constantly feeling survival emotions of lack which include lack of time, lack of money, lack of love, lack of happiness, and lack of energy, we end up feeling like we must rush. We must beat the clock. We must get as much done as we possibly can. Then we just end up tired, frustrated, and disappointed because we didn't accomplish a darn thing.

The best way that I have found to battle my inability to stay present is to do a Tapping Meditation daily. I find that calm, safe place where I know I can make better decisions. I can plan my day out and prioritize it. The second way that I have been able to get myself to use this healing insight in a beneficial way is by telling myself, "I am only doing this right now." I repeat this which helps me reframe my mind and realize that I don't need to be thinking about anything else. I don't need to be trying to do even one more thing while I am focusing on that task.

This healing insight has been very helpful in my life because it has made me slow down. I know that it's okay to just focus on one thing. To feel competent; to feel pleased with the tasks that I do complete throughout my day. This healing insight has shown me that when you're focused, you can experience flow. Flow is when you are so productive that the ease of accomplishing tasks is remarkable.

This healing insight has assisted me to achieve that state of flow to be able to develop this 70-Day Course for you. It has also helped me to focus on taking care of myself. I can give myself permission to have that time in the morning to meditate. To have that time in the morning to practice yoga. Or to exercise to prepare my mind, body, soul, and spirit for the day, and for the tasks ahead.

This healing insight has been at times extremely difficult for me to make a part of my daily life. But I appreciate it because it has allowed me to nurture myself and to not feel guilty about the self-care that I take time for each day! My goal is to help you comprehend how this healing insight can support your new healthy lifestyle, by providing you with the knowledge of how your conscious mind works, so you can use it to live your full life!

Healing Insight 46: The only way to get success is to change.

The Magic of Thinking Big, David J. Schwartz

This healing insight was revealed to me in the book *The Magic of Thinking Big* by David Schwartz. This book helps you move beyond that smallness of your mind, the self-limiting beliefs that hold you back! All the thought leaders agree on this healing insight and for good reason. It makes perfect sense that to succeed you must change. But I didn't realize to what degree I would have to change. Sure, I figured I have to change a few habits. I'll have to add some more physical activity into my life. I'll have to change the way I eat. But what I didn't realize is that I was going to have to change every aspect of my being to make those changes. In my body and in my life. These changes started with detoxing my mind, body, soul, and spirit. Not only from food not serving me but thoughts, emotions, memories, events, and people.

This process of change included releasing and processing emotion, thoughts, and any events that had held me back and kept me stuck. This change meant I would have to adopt a new mindset and reprogram my mind. To create new beliefs and a new perspective on how to make my goals a reality. I had to learn that physical activity was a huge part of this change because it helps improve your mood, decrease your stress level, increase your strength, increase your endurance, improve your energy level, and increase your level of alertness. I also learned that we change at a cellular level. So why not change at every other level to maximize for a full life?

Dr. Joe Dispenza explains the process as having to change the habit of being yourself and just becoming a new person. Essentially that's what I wanted. That's what I needed, and that's what I continue to work on as I follow this path of self-development.

I didn't realize that this change was not always as easy as it sounds. But I remind myself of the day that I walked into the living room and exclaimed to my husband, "I hate my life and who I have become!" I use this as a motivator to push me forward, especially on the most difficult days. I am just so fortunate that my family has been supportive. My oldest son is my inspiration! He constantly challenges me to read more books. He invites me to take self-development courses with him. He calls me daily so that we can exchange our insight and process what we have learned. My youngest son has been an amazing resource to me! I enjoy lunchtime when we read physical books together. I am blessed with my husband's support. He listens to all the new concepts that I am learning. Even if I might not be explaining them just right; he allows me to share these ideas with him by either reading physical books, listening to audiobooks, or watching videos during dinner time.

As a family, we are dedicated to this change. As a mother, I have decided that it is my responsibility to make this change. Not only for myself but also for my marriage, to help my children to change those old programs and false beliefs that I helped cement in their brains. I am inspired to keep going! To continue making changes so that I can pass this information on to my grandchildren. I want them to have the right programs from the beginning. So they don't have to feel hopeless. So they don't have to feel unworthy of love. So they don't have to neglect their true self. My hope is that they can live a full life. So they don't have to wander aimlessly without purpose. Questioning why they are on Earth.

I know this may sound mushy. But I realize how profound this change must be to live a full life! My goal is to share with you these healing insights to teach you the techniques, to help you, to guide you, and to support you. I want you to realize that all of this is possible. Even if at times it is challenging to make these changes to such a degree. It is well worth it! You are worth it! You can live big! You have the potential to live the life that you dreamed of when you were a child. That big life you envisioned when you were developing your character, your interests, and your goals!

Here is a bit more insight to help you make those changes that you are striving for. Did you know that the mind is easily persuaded when in the alpha (or sleepy) state of consciousness? The brain also loves to be entertained. This is why you enjoy TV, a movie, and time on social media. Plus, the brain releases hormones like dopamine during pleasurable experiences. This keeps you coming back for more. Meditation is beneficial because it places you in an alpha state of consciousness. Meditation primes your mind to change programs. "The best time to meditate is either within one hour of waking up or one hour before you go to sleep," according to Dr. Joe Dispenza.

So, entertain your brain with knowledge, with books, with wisdom, with healing insight. Do it at the times that support your ability to absorb new information. Remember that reading books releases serotonin, a natural mood stabilizer and the main hormone of happiness. Entertain your brain with these healthy activities. Like meditation and reading rather than being persuaded by all the false information that the media produces. I share this information with you so that you can use it to your advantage. Give your brain what it needs so you can be successful!

Healing Insight 47: I'm proud of you!

Dr. Jain, San Tan Allergy & Asthma

This healing insight touched my heart and inspired me to continue my journey to make the drastic changes that I needed to make to heal. When I met Dr. Jain, I was at the end of my rope. I had to switch providers because my insurance no longer had a contract with my other allergist. My primary physician advised me to get a second opinion from an allergist regarding the nasal surgery. I was hoping Dr. Jain could guide me to decide if I needed a referral to an ENT (ear, nose, and throat specialist) to determine if I had fungus in my nose.

My fatigue was unbearable along with my pain. I had just started on my journey with the 10-Day Detox Diet and The Tapping Solution Tapping Meditations. I still had not realized the power of positive thinking and using it in my favor. As I mentioned to you in Healing Insight 1, I am very thorough about informing new providers of my symptoms, conditions, and medications. I also provide any imaging or lab results if possible. So, when I showed up in Dr. Jain's office with a stack of medical records, I got his attention. I basically told him that I was at my wit's end. I didn't know, exactly, what the biggest contributor was to my situation. My system was so wiped out from being sick and tired that I was simply sick and tired of it all!

I was hoping that he would give me some guidance. He reviewed the stack of medical records as quickly as possible. Bless his heart. He was infuriated when he realized that the surgery I was scheduled for the next morning was absolutely not going to help my symptoms. He informed me that it was inappropriate for the medical conditions that I had. He told me, "If you were my wife, my daughter, or my mother I would tell you the same thing. Don't have the surgery!" He assured me he would contact the ENT that recommended the surgery to inform him of his concerns. I felt a sense of relief because I was so confused at the time. I didn't want another surgery, but I didn't know how to go about it. I was desperate. I just wanted relief from all the sinus pressure, pain, and congestion that I had been having since April of that year.

So, a year later when I returned to Dr. Jain he told me, "I'm proud of you." I was a bit shocked by his words of praise. I felt so proud of myself. I don't think I had felt self-pride about anything in several years. It was nice to know that others were seeing the improvements. I was not sure that these improvements were even possible. This beautiful gift of love gave me the confidence to continue making lifestyle changes. His praise also helped me to become my own best friend. I was able to cheer myself on from that day forward!

I had improved my liver enzymes. The results were normal. I was no longer taking sertraline, pregabalin, and several of the stomach medications that I had been on. I was able to breathe and was feeling better. Dr. Jain pointed out that difficulty breathing can cause extreme fatigue. I hadn't even considered this as a likely reason contributing to my fatigue. I highlight the connection to fatigue because you may need a specialist that you wouldn't automatically consider. So, share every symptom that you experience with your medical team.

As I look back, I smile. I feel such great admiration for Dr. Jain. I think of James Van Praagh's words in his energy clearing meditation: "Everyone you meet, you change them and they change you. It is not by chance that you meet them, it is meant to be." I am so glad that I have been blessed with Dr. Jain being placed in my path. Of course, I was heartbroken that I had to switch allergists, to begin with. I lost the awesome physician assistant that was able to see the hope in me. She got me started on this journey in the first place.

But I knew I was in great care! I knew that this was a medical provider that would become a strong team player on my journey back to health! He is open-minded when I ask him for alternative treatment. He is always encouraging when I want to try something new. I hope to help you realize that there are individuals that are truly in the right position. They are in the correct profession. Their heart is where it should be. They are not afraid to help and give guidance, so you can live your full life!

Healing Insight 48: Turn your expectations into appreciations!

Awaken the Giant Within, Tony Robbins

Another awesome concept from Tony Robbins! I hope to meet him someday. Until then, I will continue to follow him because he has given me so many blessings without even realizing his reach. This is a tremendously strong healing insight! It is an insight that will make you dig deep into your soul and connect with your spirit. It can be one of the most difficult to carry out. I say this because of the fact that we are so hard on ourselves by default, we tend to have so many negative thoughts. Remember, our subconscious mind runs the show the majority of the day. That is why this healing insight will force you into the present moment to be aware and to be conscious.

What is meant by this healing insight? It simply means to stop expecting and start appreciating! I will give you some examples of how this works. As I've mentioned, I have the need to help others especially when something as great as Tapping Meditation has helped me. I didn't realize it was not my job to change others. It was only my job to love them. So, I was always expecting my family to automatically apply what I was applying to my life. These expectations came out as nagging, as griping, as grouchiness, as persisting, as pestering, as pushy, as judgmental and controlling. I didn't understand this healing insight and didn't even realize it I was causing friction with those I loved.

How do you turn expectations into appreciations? By being grateful! Gratitude will elevate you to feel appreciation for even the smallest things. Yes, sometimes it has to be the smallest of things that you have to be grateful for. Because sometimes there's not that much progress or that much that you can see. Sometimes it is hard to realize what you should be grateful for.

Here is an example. In the beginning, I would express my desire for my husband to join me in a Tapping Meditation. When he didn't, I continued my attempt to influence him rather than being grateful for the fact that he was open to at least listening to how 'Tapping' worked and how it was helping me. I should have just been grateful for his support. This healing insight goes back to the magnetizing energy cycle of the Law of Attraction. Use this concept to attract what you want into your life!

Here is another example about me. I should have been grateful for the progress I had made which had allowed me to be less reactive to situations of stress. Instead of being hard on myself, I should have been grateful. Even though I wasn't totally able to control myself, I was able to make a responsible decision when I lashed out with words. I should have just been grateful that I didn't throw something across the room. I should have been grateful that I at least know now that I have the ability to respond and to realize that I wasn't going to react any further. As you can see, this has been a great challenge for me.

I am so thankful that I was able to learn these techniques from the many self-development courses I have immersed myself in. Also, I am pleased that these techniques are now part of my coping skills toolbox. I hope that I can help you understand that gratitude is the ultimate way to achieve the state of mind to balance your energy system. Gratitude is the way to make these changes in your life. By staying grateful, you can create a space to heal! So you can create the life you deserve!

We tend to forget all the big and small blessings we have on a daily basis. Much of what we should be counting as blessings we take for granted. We expect that we should have many things like running water, electricity, and air conditioning. These are huge blessings! Not to mention all the little things that we don't realize we should continually be grateful for. Such as our ability to give hugs to our loved ones and smiles that we get in return. The warmth of the sunshine even if we can just sit by the window. See all of the blessings that are around you every day. Learn how to turn your expectations into appreciations!

Healing Insight 49: You can invite abundance into your life.

Annual Tapping World Summit, Carol Look, *The Yes Code*

This healing insight caught me off guard. I had already heard about detoxing your mind, body, and spirit. Processing and releasing emotions not serving you. Creating a positive mindset, the need to reprogram your mind. How exercise and physical activity was so beneficial. But when I heard, "You can invite abundance into your life," I was baffled. I thought, wait a minute…isn't that what a positive mindset is for?

This healing insight was an awakening that I needed! Carol Look's "Using EFT to Invite Abundance Tapping Meditation" script totally spiked my interest. I was all ears, or should I say all eyes. As I read the script I was in awe! I thought this is amazing! What an awesome concept. You can process and release emotions not serving you. Plus, invite abundance into your life! How can this get any better?

This script laid it all out for me. It had elements of what all the other thought leaders that I follow emphasize. Elements like, "Raise your vibration." "Look forward to exciting results." "Feel the vibrational shift and power already!" "Bring more of what you want into your life!" "Tap every day to release your blocks to attracting abundance." Again, I was picking up on a pattern, a system, a blueprint.

I felt as if the handbook to life had just been handed to me. Everything was coming together in my mind on how to live a full life. This was the icing on the cake! She spelled it out in these phrases. "Be so specific with my invitation to the Universe." "Send abundance invitations." "Make the time and effort to invite abundance in." "Feel more aligned with abundance already!" Another 'aha' moment for me! I felt lucky! How could I not feel this way? I had the blueprint. Now, I just needed to invite abundance in literally!

This stroke of luck came via email once again from good old Nick Ortner at TheTappingSolution.com. It was truly a gift to me. It gave me more fuel. So of course, I used the script and began 'Tapping' to invite abundance into my life! I still feel so blessed when I think about the healing insight that this Tapping Meditation script gave me.

I hope that I am expressing how important this healing insight is in this process. It is essentially the bonus that you can apply to your daily life; it adds so much control to the idea of using the Law of Attraction to turn your thoughts into reality. It gives you such a wonderful feeling of empowerment! There's no way you can feel like a victim once you know that, "You can invite abundance into your life!" Seriously!

I feel refreshed just sharing this healing insight with you! Because it reminds me of all the higher-level emotions I was showered with. The aim of this healing insight is to elevate your ability to bring all the goodness into your life. Know that by adding this bit of inspiration to your effort, it will pay off! I want to help you learn how to use every level of these techniques to bring you health, wealth, love, and happiness!

Healing Insight 50: Gratitude is on the same vibration as abundance.

Annual Tapping World Summit, Mary Morrissey, MaryMorrissey.com, *Turning Possibilities into Realities*

This healing insight means that when you are in a state of gratitude, then you are vibrating your energy to be abundant. So, gratitude attracts abundance! I just kept thinking, wow, I guess I should be grateful! It seems to work. But how do you automatically go from being angry, disgusted, hurt, ashamed, guilty, and sad to switching on the gratitude mindset? It doesn't happen overnight. But it is possible.

When you know all of these healing insights and how the body and the brain work, you can do this! How can you manipulate your body and brain to overcome your situation? You can turn on the gratitude switch! This is not just expressing that you are grateful. You can say it all day long. You can write it and fill a million gratitude journals. But you must feel it! Send out that positive gratitude to the energy field. Take action on it! See it. To see it is to be grateful for those blessings before they have even happened, so that you can attract what you were grateful for back to you, like a magnet!

I will be honest with you. It takes time. It takes practice. It takes dedication. It takes will. But if I can do it, so can you! If you remember, I mentioned that I had been angry since I was a young child. That's all I knew. So even though I consider myself optimistic, I didn't feel those higher-level emotions. Because I didn't feel how it would be if those things that I desired had already happened. That's the secret! Then I couldn't make that positive cycle work for me. To deepen your comprehension of the Law of Attraction, add *The Secret* by Rhonda Byrne to your reading list.

I didn't have this knowledge of what it took. Even though I used the Law of Attraction throughout my life, I didn't know what it was. I didn't know what I was truly doing. I didn't know the process involved. So, I didn't hone this skill. I didn't use it consistently so that it could become a constant in my life because I was in the stress response cycle and that state of mind; experiencing survival emotions of unworthiness, anger, fear, frustration, resentment, hate, and lack. I was using the Law of Attraction—the *negative* Law of Attraction cycle! I couldn't see or use it to my advantage. I was drawing the negative cycle to me without even realizing what I was doing.

I'm sorry that I must repeat this so many times. But I need you to understand how critical this is. We don't question the Law of Gravity. When a ball gets thrown in the air it comes down, right? So why do we question the Law of Attraction? Positive attracts positive and negative attracts negative. That's it.

I want this to become a consistent process for you. Remember, repetition and energy psychology are two ways that change old programs. If you can combine these two—Tapping Meditations can change your mindset. You can reprogram your mind!

I understand how extremely difficult it is to stay grateful, to see the positive. To find reasons to feel better. It's hard to completely feel and believe that you can experience the higher-level emotions of joy, empowerment, safety, calm, love, and forgiveness, but they must be felt so you can attract your health back to you. It is possible! I want this for you because I didn't get the message! I suffered needlessly! I don't want anyone to suffer the way I did! The formula is simple!

Apply this knowledge to your life every day. Use Tapping Meditations to elevate you into a state of 'super learning,' so that you can switch to an abundant mindset and learn how to use gratitude to stay on the same vibration as abundance. Abundance is within your reach! Grab it and never look back! Use it and learn how to maximize for a full life! Learn how to create a space to heal! Learn how to live a pain-free life and love every minute of it!

Healing Insight 51: Always add "or something better" to your goals.

8th Annual Tapping World Summit, Mary Ayers, TappingIntoAction.com

This healing insight was an absolute blessing from the 8th Annual Tapping World Summit, another free online event that I encourage you to participate in. Not only do you get access to new Tapping Meditations, you also get to listen to expert interviews from other providers in the 'Tapping' world. It is so uplifting to see the different fields of practice that Tapping Meditation is applied to. There are doctors, marriage counselors, addiction counselors, trauma counselors, PTSD counselors, life coaches, financial coaches, and of course EFT Tapping practitioners.

Plus, you also learn new ways to use the Tapping Meditation Process. Such as just starting at the eyebrow point and not using the setup phrases. Or you can select one acupressure point to stimulate during the meditation. Much like we've done with just the collarbone point or the Spirit Gate 7 at the side of the wrist. This event is so valuable to anyone just learning about Tapping Meditation. It is also great for anyone who has been using it for a while. Either way, you will learn a tremendous amount of new insight!

When this healing insight was explained yet again, I had an 'aha' moment. I thought, *Crazy! You can send out abundance invitations plus ask for 'something better'! How can this be?* This concept had me so intrigued that I made note of it in my War Room Journal, immediately! I started adding this to my journal when I listed my gratitude for future blessings. I thought, what could it hurt, right? If it works, it's a bonus!

Once I started reading Dr. Joe Dispenza's books there was mention of this concept again. In the book *You Are the Placebo: Making Your Mind Matter* there is a story about a woman who had started using Dr. Dispenza's meditation technique. To make a long story short, she started living and making decisions through an abundant mindset. One day she decided to buy a lottery ticket. She thought about the money she needed to cover her bills. Of course, she won exactly what she needed to cover her bills, which was $56,000. She had been instructed to add 'or something better' to the end of her desire, but she didn't do it. She was amazed that she had won exactly the amount she needed. She said, "Next time I will add 'or something better.'"

Amazing! It really is worth adding 'or something better' to your goals and desires. I know it may seem hard to believe that this simple concept can make a difference and can cause such huge results. But you must remember what you are really causing because you are practicing an abundant mindset. The feelings, the confidence, the belief automatically pulls that desire, that goal, 'or something better' toward you. This is hard to understand when you are operating in a scarcity mindset. Just know that it is possible. Apply it as a Band-Aid—why not, right? What's the worst that could happen? You might just win a lottery ticket to cover exactly what your bills are. What's the best that could happen? Who knows? Find out by adding 'or something better' to all your goals and desires.

I understand how this information can be misunderstood. That is why this book includes my 5-Step Process. Detox, releasing emotion, mindset, reprogramming your mind, and exercise/physical activity. Believe it or not, these steps will help you to nurture your mind, body, soul, and spirit to become aligned with an abundant mindset. Don't just take my word for it. Use the power you have. Make things happen through thought alone. Send out such positive energy that you can feel it before it has even happened. Take action to cause this reality to come true. Who knows, maybe you will get something even better!

My goal is to help you realize that operating from an abundant mindset leads to more abundance in every area of your life. Do you consider yourself an open-minded person? I want to help you to be open-minded enough to understand these concepts, to be inspired by these healing insights that inspired me, to turn hope into action! I want to help you feel how it feels to have health, wealth, love, and happiness before it has taken place. To do this you must totally surrender. While you embrace your body to reach total health, forgive your mind to accomplish endless wealth, love your soul to achieve true love, and honor your spirit to create pure happiness.

I want to help you learn how to cheer yourself on. I want to show you how to believe in yourself. I want to help you realize that these concepts are real. I want to help you understand that no matter how silly these concepts seem, once they are applied to your life the results will astound you! Finally, I want to help you learn my 5-Step Process so that you can gain this knowledge, apply it to your life, and enjoy the benefits of making decisions with an abundant mindset. To live the life you deserve 'or something better'!

Healing Insight 52: Our mind is our single most powerful asset.

Rich Dad Poor Dad, Robert Kiyosaki

When I read this healing insight, I figured, well Robert Kiyosaki must be referring to his concept, "Great opportunities are not seen with your eyes... they are seen with your mind." I thought that makes sense because he's talking about financial education. Once you understand how money flows in and out then you can start to see with your mind. I also thought he was talking about how the mind can help us be financially savvy; when you are knowledgeable about the flow of cash you learn how to hold on to money, rather than just spending it.

This healing insight went beyond the obvious.

As I kept reading, I realized that Mr. Kiyosaki was on to something. Not only was he financially literate but he had also mastered the cash flow game in his own life. He could see money with his mind. He certainly knew how to hold on to it or invest his money. Rather than just spending his money on items that end up being liabilities rather than assets. But he also was talking about how powerful the mind is. The ability we have to control our lives at every level.

He knew that you need the right mindset to release thoughts not serving you, and change old programs. He knew that you had to focus your attention and put all your energy into mastering your goals. He knew how to harness the power of the Law of Attraction. He was spreading the word in his own, subtle way; or maybe not-so-subtle way. However you choose to perceive his books. Either way, he was shedding light on the fact that your mind could be fueled with positive thoughts, positive feelings, and strong actions to improve your effort and draw positive results to you.

Mr. Kiyosaki not only shared his financial savvy in his books, he also shared his upbringing and how mindset was a huge factor. He showed how his biological father and his mentor had such different lives. Mr. Kiyosaki had an amazing mind at a very young age. He was very observant and driven. So driven that he chose to change his mindset and reprogram his mind. He did that by asking his mentor to help him. I don't mean he didn't love his biological father. He just didn't want his dad's lifestyle. More so, he didn't want to be stuck in a scarcity mindset. He had seen how the abundant mindset could propel his ability, how it could open the possibilities in his life to such a degree to show him that there was nothing that could hold him back from being successful.

It was amazing to me to see all the differences when comparing each mindset! I also become aware of how easy or difficult it made the lifestyles of his biological father and mentor. I noticed so much of my own upbringing in the mindset of his biological father. I too had been programmed with a scarcity mindset, since I was a child. I felt sad because I felt at such a disadvantage. But not for long because I felt the hope that Mr. Kiyosaki shared! I could see that our mind is so powerful. I believe mindset and programs can be changed. Once you see the possibilities, then your mind can make it happen! The distinction that Mr.

Kiyosaki highlighted between an abundant mindset and a scarcity mindset was a huge blessing. I didn't even realize two mindsets existed.

Once I realized the mindsets were so different, I was interested in how I could become an abundant thinker. Knowing that an abundant mindset can work for you in all areas of your life for health, wealth, love, and happiness kept my attention. Of course, I needed help with these areas at the time. So, I thought might as well try to implement these ideas. Why not? It worked for Mr. Kiyosaki! It surely can work for me, right?

I don't know that I truly understood what I was reading when I read Mr. Kiyosaki's book *Rich Dad Poor Dad*. But by the time I read *Rich Dad's Cashflow Quadrant: Rich Dad's Guide to Financial Freedom*, I had some experience with his *Cashflow* board game via the app. I was beginning to understand how this abundant mindset could help you attract anything. I didn't comprehend the weight of this healing insight until I started following Dr. Bruce Lipton. When I started following Dr. Joe Dispenza, I finally understood.

I share this healing insight with you because it is true—your mind is so powerful. It's the most powerful asset that you have! I want to help you learn how to use your mind to your advantage, so you can see the possibilities! So you can maximize for your full life!

Healing Insight 53: To improve your marriage, it is better to improve yourself.

Rich Dad's Cashflow Quadrant: Rich Dad's Guide to Financial Freedom, Robert Kiyosaki

Robert Kiyosaki finished explaining this healing insight in his book, *Rich Dad's Cashflow Quadrant: Rich Dad's Guide to Financial Freedom*. He said, "Don't work on the other person, work on your thoughts about the other person." This healing insight was super hard for me to accept, to comprehend, and to apply to my life because I had come from a scarcity mindset. I never thought I had enough. I was stuck feeling survival emotions of lack and victimization. I didn't want to believe that I had to improve myself to have a better marriage. It was so much easier to blame my husband. That's what you do when you are experiencing victimization. You make every excuse possible. You blame everyone else instead of looking inward and realizing that you need to make some changes.

So many thought leaders are saying the same thing but in a little different way. Think about Tony Robbins' quote, "Turn your expectations into appreciations." Many times, the expectations we have are inappropriate, so we place blame and judgment on ourselves and others. We are not focusing on the blessings or appreciating what is already working in our relationship. We only focus on what is not working. Remember what Dr. Joe Dispenza said: "Wherever you place your attention is where you place your energy." It's no wonder we are stuck in this scarcity mindset, swimming in survival emotions. All our energy is being placed on the negative.

Think of it like this. If you blame your spouse for everything and feel that they must change but they blame you for everything and feel that you must change, but nobody is willing to change, you're still doing the same thing. So, the situation is still the same. You are still thinking the same thoughts. You're still feeling the same survival emotions. You are still acting or reacting the same way. Nothing is changing because no one has taken responsibility to change. Therefore, couples continue to have arguments over the same thing throughout their time together.

I did not want to accept the fact that maybe my relationship was strained because of me. But the Law of Attraction stands to prove my point. James Van Praagh describes the Law of Attraction as, "like attracts like." If I am focusing on the negative, I am attracting the negative. If I can focus on the positive, then I will attract the positive. To attract the positive, I need to place my attention and my energy on changing things that I can control and that I can change. Remember, it's not your job to change others, you can only love them. We can only change ourselves.

This was a hard pill to swallow. To look in the mirror and accept the fact that I was the reason my life was such a mess. This was one of the most difficult things that I had to accept and forgive myself for. But I had to see the dirt before I could clean it up, right? I never said this would be easy. I just said these concepts are simple, almost common sense. But to apply them to your life takes action, dedication, and accepting the realization that you have to take responsibility for your own well-being. This is the only way you can create a sense of balance to access your ability to see your full potential. The only way that you can help yourself to be primed for success. The only way that you can truly honor your mind, body, soul, and spirit.

I applied this healing insight to my own life by doing all the activities in the self-development courses. *The Five Love Languages* by Gary Chapman was extremely helpful. First, my husband and I identified what our primary and secondary love languages were. Then I followed the guidelines of how to use the love languages to improve my ability to love my husband in his love language (words of affirmation and physical touch). It was hard to not use my love language (acts of service and quality time). Next, I had to enlist his help to assess me monthly. He had to assess me on how I was doing with being a better partner. How I was doing loving him in his love language. The whole first month you're not allowed to request your partner to love you in your love language. No matter how deprived you feel.

I also took the extra challenge and did the six-month activity. Again, monthly assessments were required to determine how I was or was not improving. I will say that this is one of the most difficult activities I have done. I had to open myself up to the judgment of my husband. However, he was not as tough on me as I thought he would be. I think I was tougher on myself. This activity helped our relationship tremendously. I was able to release many of the thoughts, emotions, and memories that were holding me back. It also helped me to reframe the judgments, blame, and reactions I was having related to our relationship. I was able to turn my expectations into appreciations. I realized that I could focus on the positive, the blessings I already had in my marriage.

Your journey is not over when you complete this activity. The real challenge is to apply these techniques to your life, to apply these healing insights on a long-term basis. An abundant mindset will allow you to focus on the positive. The Tapping Meditation Process will let you process and release survival emotions not serving you. The repetition is what will create the healthy habits in your new amazing life! You will begin to reprogram your mind every time you apply these healing insights because you are taking action. You will use the Law of Attraction automatically when you focus on the positive. You will be given extra blessings when you remember to add 'or something better' to your intentions.

Healing Insight 54: Your conscious mind creates the thought; your subconscious mind carries it out.

The Placebo Effect, Dr. Bruce Lipton

I have mentioned this healing insight throughout this book, because it is absolutely powerful! It still astonishes me! I mentioned to you that I didn't start connecting and understanding what the Law of Attraction was until I started following Dr. Bruce Lipton. He does such a wonderful job explaining why things are important. Exactly how they work and why they work. He gives such great descriptions and comparisons. You are not left with any questions. You are just left with curiosity, wonder, excitement, and motivation.

He not only helps you realize the science involved in the Law of Attraction, but also helps you realize the connection between spirit and how spirituality drives this force. I was surprised when Dr. Lipton admitted that as a scientist he found spirituality. I thought that was amazing! It made me more curious about this entire concept of having two minds that operate as a team. We must understand how they work so that we can use them to enhance our lives, to improve our well-being, to truly be happy. To learn that wealth is not just money. It is health, wealth, love, and happiness.

With this knowledge, that the conscious mind creates the plan and the subconscious mind carries it out, there are no limits to what we can accomplish. This is not a question of will it work. This is proof of how it works. If you can truly comprehend this healing insight, then you can realize that you have the power to create the life you deserve. You have the power as Dr. Lipton says, "to have heaven on Earth." This was so appealing to me since I had been living in hell. That was how I described the year 2012 to my physician assistant when I went in for a doctor visit. I told him, "The last year of my life has been pure hell!" I was putting it mildly.

I wondered if this is truly how our minds work. If I created this hell that I'd been living in, then I can create happiness, health, and why not heaven? I hope that you are starting to see how these healing insights came into play. Either simultaneously or to support one another as I was on this journey to heal. It seemed like I was discovering more and more ways of how I could help myself. How I could have always helped myself if I would have known this as a child or even as a young adult. As I learned these healing insights, I began to comprehend them as one healing insight would help me see how the others worked. I was blown away by how forceful they were!

I began to believe in myself. I began to believe in the process. I began to believe in the Law of Attraction. I began to believe that I could truly be healthy again—once I discovered that I could be happy, and I learned how to forgive. I was having more and more positive thoughts, feelings, and actions. Changes were taking place in my body as well as in my life. I was excited! I felt alive! I felt empowered! I felt so blessed; I was feeling the love and the forgiveness that I needed to feel from myself many, many years ago! I felt capable of taking on this abundant mindset. I knew it was going to help me! To create a space to heal! So, that I could take back my health, take control of my life, and find relief!

I was feeling stronger physically, emotionally, mentally, and spiritually. I felt like I was truly connecting with spirit, to my true self. I felt like I was a new person, a better person, a happier person. The person that I wanted to be! I wasn't just imagining these changes. My lab results were proof. My mood was better, my energy level was better, my pain was disappearing. I had been in misery for so long that I could hardly believe how I was feeling. I had so much relief I felt so safe, so calm, so confident, and so happy, I had made so many changes with my diet, my lifestyle, and my emotional well-being, and I wasn't the only one that was noticing my improved condition. My medical providers were noticing it too. My family was not only seeing the physical improvements, they were feeling the emotional and spiritual improvements as well.

I'm excited to help you comprehend these healing insights to the highest level that you can. I want to show you how you can create a space to heal! How you can maximize for a full life! How you can truly have heaven on Earth! Follow these steps. Now that you know how your mind and body work, use them to create the life you deserve!

Activity:

"Law of Attraction in Action!"

Instructions:

- List positive and negative thoughts you created in the past and the results you attracted.

"Law of Attraction in Action!" Activity Sheet

Positive Thought	Positive Result	Negative Thought	Negative Result

Daily Challenge:

Turn Hope into Action!

"Rinse & Repeat!"

- Repeat the "Law of Attraction in Action" today!

- Create a positive thought to attract positive results into your life!

Reminder: You always knew how to use the Law of Attraction! You just didn't have a name for it.

Healing Insight 55: I am the placebo.

You Are the Placebo, Dr. Joe Dispenza

Dr. Joe Dispenza's concept 'you are the placebo' simply means that whatever you believe in will heal you. His explanation, research, and data supporting the fact that 'you are the placebo' is absolutely fascinating! It will grab your attention! It will make you sit at the edge of your chair! It will make you yearn for the healing that you thought was impossible! As I mentioned in Healing Insight 54, I finally fully understood and made the connection of how powerful the mind is! Everything I had been reading connected my understanding about the 'placebo effect' from Dr. Bruce Lipton. His definition of the 'placebo effect' is positive thoughts that generate positive effects.

When I realized Dr. Dispenza was going to be at the Hay House U Live 2017 Conference, I was ecstatic! Not only was Nick Ortner going to be there from TheTappingSolution.com, but now I could see Dr. Dispenza as well—sweet! When I looked at the itinerary, I felt sad because both Nick Ortner and Dr. Dispenza were on the same day. I signed up for the volunteer work program; the agreement was to volunteer one day. The other day I was able to participate in any of the speakers that were available. Once I knew that I was assigned to James Van Praagh I had to make my decision. I was torn because I truly do love Dr. Joe Dispenza's work. TheTappingSolution.com, specifically Nick Ortner, has been so instrumental in my healing process from the beginning but I already knew that Tapping Meditation worked. I was so curious about Dr. Dispenza's meditation technique especially since I had just fully comprehended how powerful the mind and the body connection is. So, I chose to go see Dr. Joe Dispenza. (I did get to meet Nick Ortner at the book signing, so I didn't totally miss out.)

The month before we went to the Hay House U Live 2017 Conference, I started meditating using Dr. Joe Dispenza's meditation technique. He has pre-recorded guided meditations to help you meditate. My goal was to decrease or stop more of the prescription medications that I was taking. In the month that I started meditating before the conference, I was able to stop taking my muscle relaxants for muscle spasms related to fibromyalgia. I had already started reducing them and now I was able to just meditate the spasms away! I have always 'Tapped' on my favorite acupressure point while meditating. But in Dr. Dispenza's March 2017 newsletter, he featured Dr. Bruce Lipton's article, which reminded me that 'Tapping' is one of the four ways to reprogram the subconscious mind. So, I don't forget to 'Tap' during every meditation!

After the conference, I focused on my bladder prescription medications which included a muscle relaxant for the bladder and a vaginal suppository for the pain due to pelvic floor tension myalgia. During that same time, I was using Dr. Dispenza's meditation technique to attract sales for my son's e-commerce business. It seemed to be working! I was excited to take on my bladder prescription medications! The only thing is Dr. Joe Dispenza warns you that when you decide to stay conscious and take over your body again instead of letting the subconscious programs run your body, your body continues to try to be your brain. He says that your body will reject the fact that your brain is now in control again. So, your symptoms will increase. Your critical voice will tell you why you shouldn't be making these changes in your life. Boy, that's exactly what happened. My pelvic floor had spasms for two and a half weeks straight! I was wiped out mentally, physically, emotionally, and spiritually.

I thought, *Damn! I don't know how much longer I can hold out.* But I started thinking about how I felt when I meditated, and those sales came in for my son's e-commerce business. Dr. Dispenza says to remember those higher-level emotions; once you learn that process you can apply it to anything! So, I started remembering how I felt. I felt safe. I felt calm. I felt comfort. I felt relief. I felt love. I felt forgiveness. I felt self-love and self-forgiveness. I felt empowered, connected, whole. I felt oneness with my true self. I felt grateful, blessed, and thankful that I had learned this meditation technique. I just kept feeling those emotions again and again as I meditated.

In Dr. Dispenza's book, *Breaking the Habit of Being Yourself: How to Lose Your Mind and Create a New One*, he further explains it like this: "If you can mentally rehearse the desired experience by thought alone, you will experience the emotions of that event before it is physically manifested. Now you are moving into a new state of being, because your mind and body are working as one when you begin to feel like some future potential reality is happening to you. In the moment when you are focusing on it, you are rewriting your automatic habits, attitudes, and other unwanted subconscious programs. When you meditate and connect to something greater, you can create and then memorize such coherence between your thoughts and feelings that nothing in your outer reality—no thing, no person, no condition at any place or time—could move you from that level of energy. Now you are mastering your environment, your body, and time."

I want to help you feel those higher-level emotions so you can master this technique. Remember, you can't just have a positive thought. You must have a positive thought while experiencing higher-level emotions such as gratitude, joy, acceptance, service, and love. Once you realize that this is the secret to sending out abundant invitations to the universe, your healing is a question of when not if! As I grasped the steps in this meditation technique, I realized there are three major parts. 1. Your thoughts have to matter to send out positive energy. 2. You have to make your thoughts and emotions match by surrendering your mind, body, soul, and spirit. 3. You must take action to attract positive effects back to you! Please allow me to guide you through the process so you can create a pain-free life and love every minute of it!

Activity:

"What's Your Placebo?"

Instructions:

- List 5 items that you believe are your placebo (medication, natural remedies, exercise/physical activity, etc.)

- List the result you get.

- List how soon you feel the results.

"What's Your Placebo" Activity Sheet

Placebo	Result	How Soon

Daily Challenge:

Turn Hope into Action!

"New State of Being!"

- Move into a new state of being today!

- Pick a placebo from the "What's Your Placebo" Activity Sheet.

- Use the emotions you feel when that placebo takes effect to make your thoughts and emotions match.

- Allow your mind and body to work as one!

- 'Tap' on your favorite acupressure point to reprogram your subconscious mind!

Healing Insight 56: Believe in pronoia.

The Little Book of Gratitude: Create a life of happiness and wellbeing by giving thanks, Dr. Robert A. Emmons

I have always prided myself in knowing many definitions of words, having a large vocabulary due to the number of books I read. But this one term, I had never heard of. I had never come across it. I had no idea what the definition was. This term has fascinated me so much that I think of it on a daily basis. I stumbled upon this brilliant term in a book that my youngest son bought me called *The Little Book of Gratitude*. The author, Dr. Robert A. Emmons, is a professor of psychology and the director of the Gratitude Lab at the University of California. I said, "What? A gratitude lab!" Yes, they study gratitude to find out if it can make you feel happier. Guess what? The results showed that being grateful does make you happier! I was amazed because it hadn't even crossed my mind that gratitude would be part of a research study.

Pronoia means a belief that people conspire to do good especially in the goodwill of others. I said, "Wow!" *Now I understand why all of the thought leaders are trying to get their message out to the masses.* They have a belief in pronoia. They truly want to share their message for the good of others. I felt exceptionally blessed as I thought of 'the term of the day' so to speak. I shared it with my family. This healing insight inspired me to realize that I was so fortunate that all of these magnificent people had come into my life throughout this journey. I was beginning to believe it was meant to be.

I needed to learn the lessons that they were sharing. I needed to understand these healing insights, to be able to apply them to my life so I could create a space to heal. Even though I didn't meet these people in person, I felt their energy, their love, their forgiveness, and the pronoia. As well as their ability to see the possibility in all of us. I could feel their deep desire to help others. I felt it in their books, emails, recipes, videos, online summits, webinars, and courses.

Once I learned this new term, I understood what was behind their need to share their story, their message. I understood how deep from the goodness of their heart they wanted to help others learn this message. So others could learn to heal their mind, their body, their soul, and their spirit. This healing insight really helped me to understand how I have been blessed with so many mentors and they don't even know me. I appreciate all of the thought leaders that have made such a huge impact on my life. How the healthcare providers in my life have become such great team members, as well.

I wanted to share this healing insight with my mother-in-law because she has been struggling with a diagnosis that has no cure and very little treatment options. Even though it was a gift from my son, he understood that I needed to share this book with her. I finished the book in September of 2017 as we were driving to see my husband's family for the weekend. I took pictures of the pages of the activities that I had not yet finished. I knew that every one of these activities would heal me just a little bit more, that the activities would help me make these connections stronger, to help me reprogram my mind with this new belief. I knew that pronoia needed to be more than just a new term or a new definition that I could pride myself in knowing. I knew that pronoia was now a new program (a new belief) that I could apply to my life.

I had discovered the higher-level emotions that these thought leaders experience. I found such love, service, joy, and happiness knowing that I could conspire to do good. Not only for myself and for my family, but also for people I don't even know. I wondered—is this the goodwill that is talked about? Is this the goodwill that is sent out? When there's nothing else for us to do but send our blessings, love, faith, and hope to others? I believed it was. I just didn't know the term for it.

This new belief has been the fuel to encourage me to see the possibilities! Not only in myself and my family, but also in you! I want to help you learn, understand, accept, and apply this new belief to your life. I want to help you see the possibilities in yourself so that you can feel rejuvenated! So you can be pain-free! So you can be calm! So you can be stress-free! So you can help yourself, heal yourself, and live your full life!

Healing Points to Treasure

1. Give yourself permission to forgive, love, and nurture yourself without holding back. Nurture your inner child to heal lifelong wounds.

2. Recognize that you are only responsible for your own happiness. This healing insight will not only heal your entire being, it will help you nurture your emotional well-being!

3. Your conscious mind can only focus on one thing. When you're focused, you can experience flow. Flow is when you are so productive that the ease of accomplishing tasks is remarkable.

4. To succeed, you must change! This process includes detox, releasing and processing emotion, a positive mindset, reprogramming your mind, and physical activity. Meditation primes your mind to change old programs.

5. The beautiful gift of love from people's words of praise will give you the confidence to continue making lifestyle changes. Also, allow yourself to feel self-pride. Cheer yourself on from this day forward!

6. Stop expecting and start appreciating! Turn expectations into appreciations by being grateful! Gratitude will elevate you to feel appreciation for even the smallest things.

7. Remember you can invite abundance into your life. This is the handbook on how to live a full life. This is the icing on the cake!

8. When you are in a state of gratitude you are vibrating your energy to be abundant. So, gratitude attracts abundance!

9. You can send out abundance invitations plus ask for 'something better'! It's a bonus!

10. Your mind is the single most powerful asset! Harness the power of the Law of Attraction to improve your effort and draw positive results to you!

11. Focus on the positive blessings that you already have in your relationships. To attract the positive, place your attention and energy on changing things you can control and can change.

12. The conscious mind creates the plan, and the subconscious mind carries it out. There are no limits to what you can accomplish!

13. 'You are the placebo' simply means that whatever you believe in will heal you. The 'placebo effect' states that positive thoughts generate positive effects.

14. Pronoia means a belief that people conspire to do good, especially in the goodwill of others. Let it be the fuel to encourage you to see the possibilities! Not only for yourself, but in others, too.

CHAPTER FIVE

Step 5 Exercise/Physical Activity: Healing Insights 57-70

Use movement to keep your energy centers (chakras) clear and moving freely. Find the little flame that hasn't burned out. Nurture it. Believe in it. Place your hope and your faith in it. Know that something good will come from it. See the possibilities!

Exercise and physical activity saved me. I lived with chronic pain day and night. Pain medications gave me little to no relief. I was at my wit's end. I promised myself in 2014 that it would be the last year that I would be in the condition I was. At that point in my life, I would have taken death as the solution to my situation. However, I was blessed with my loving family, caring medical team, and many generous personal growth and self-development mentors!

What I was about to learn about exercise and physical activity would help me understand how detrimental the chronic stress response cycle is. What I share with you will help you realize that your knowledge is inaccessible during times of stress! You will understand the powerful force habits have on your everyday life. You will understand how the lack of movement not only harms you physically but emotionally and spiritually.

This chapter will help you comprehend the meaning of overall well-being. You will understand how movement includes breathing and energy cleansing. You will discover how to believe in yourself to create a healthy lifestyle. You will be given multiple ways to add exercise and physical activity to your daily life. You will feel the hope, the healing, and the peace! You will realize your potential, so you can live your full life!

Healing Insight 57: When you're sick, your education goes out the window.

Judy Acevedo, my aunt

This healing insight came from my aunt. She is a nurse. So of course, she has a broad knowledge base for me to rely on and to use as a resource. After three of our immediate family members passed away in 2016 within a four-month span, I believe this was too much for my aunt to handle. Her sister had passed away in April. Two weeks later her father passed away. Within four months we lost our third family member, her niece, the granddaughter of my aunt that had passed away in April. I know this was difficult for my aunt especially because she lived with her father several times throughout her life. She had just recently retired to care for him when he started slowing down.

I believe my aunt was stuck in the stress response cycle, and for good reason. Bless her heart even though she's a nurse, she was also handed down poor lifestyle habits. She developed diabetes from those poor lifestyle habits. She was having issues with her diabetes when I called to check on her one day. She had been to the doctor. I asked her what was suggested. I asked her several questions that she could have or should have asked the doctor but didn't. Her comment to me was, "When you're sick, your education goes out the window."

This healing insight gave me so much relief because I had been so hard on myself. I had been thinking how stupid I had been. I am an occupational therapy assistant by trade. I have an early childhood education degree, as well. So, I have essentially studied the development of the human being from birth till death. That education has included many techniques to improve well-being and promote good health. But I just kept torturing myself, wondering why I didn't apply my knowledge to my situation, to my medical conditions, to my life.

When my aunt made this comment, I took a deep breath, and I understood. I agreed with her. I explained how she made me feel better about my own situation. This healing insight showed me I could be gentle on myself. I could observe my experiences on this journey and be kind. It allowed me to let go of the judgment that I had placed on myself for such a long time. It helped me to understand how my brain and body worked to such a deeper level. It helped me realize that when you are in the stress response cycle. You do not think clearly! You cannot think clearly!

It made me realize how stuck I had really been. I might still be stuck in the stress response cycle if I hadn't been blessed with these wonderful thought leaders, medical providers, and my family during this healing process. This healing insight has inspired me to take more action by being aware of the amount of stress in my life. It has shown me once again how detrimental the stress response cycle is when you are stuck there for a long time. It made me realize that to think clearly, I needed to be calm. To see the possibility, I needed to let go of the past. I needed to stop beating up myself. I needed to start noticing that there are physiological and biological effects caused by stress.

It's okay to be gentle. It's okay to just observe and not judge. It's okay that you didn't get the message because most of us did not. It's okay that you didn't get the right programming. You don't have to blame yourself or others. Ultimately, it is okay to love and forgive yourself. I'm not saying to just blame it on your brain and body. Even though they run old programs, false beliefs, and bad habits, they are just efficient. They take over and run on autopilot because that's their job.

What I am saying is that it is extremely important to know and understand what you are up against! Now that you have this new knowledge you can apply it to your life. You don't have to be sick! You don't have to let your education go out the window! You don't have to stay stuck in the stress response cycle! You can choose to apply these healing insights to your life by focusing your attention on the positive. That is the first step to creating a space to heal, so you can create the life you deserve!

Healing Insight 58: Take deep breaths.

Dr. Kan Yu, Western Neurology

This healing insight packs a whole lot of power! There are two healing insights within this one. Let me explain. My neurologist told me early in my journey, "Take deep breaths—you worry too much." I didn't realize until later how beneficial this healing insight truly was. Taking deep breaths calms your central nervous system. It helps you access the part of your parasympathetic nervous system which controls healing. It helps you create a space to heal. No wonder my neurologist told me this.

We don't do much deep breathing at all during the day, or even during our lifetime. If you don't practice yoga or some type of meditation technique that requires you to inhale deeply through your nose and exhale through your mouth, you're probably not in the habit of breathing deeply. It is so beneficial when you can breathe what is called a tummy breath. When the chest rises, and the tummy expands when you breathe.

The other part of this healing insight is 'you worry too much.' Think of all the times you worried about something that might happen. Now think about the result. Did it even take place the way you thought it would? If it did happen, was it as severe as you thought it would be? Your answer is probably no. That's because worry is a worthless emotion according to James Van Praagh. I wish I would have met him sooner than April 2017. I haven't been much of a worrier. But obviously, because I was stuck in the stress response cycle, I was experiencing these survival emotions which includes worry. They are a package deal, remember? I was not in control of my thoughts, emotions, actions, or reactions in my everyday life.

I had gotten in the habit of worrying without even realizing it because my subconscious was running the show. I had become a worrier. Yes, this is a bad thing. It takes your focus off the positive. It places your energy outward instead of on you. It causes you great stress and emotional pain. It keeps you stuck in the past and worried about the future. You can never be present. Worry really is an emotion that you should rid yourself of! Worry keeps you from realizing the possibilities. Worry keeps you in a scarcity mindset. Worry makes you think can't instead of how. So, then you are unable to change but to and to find a solution. Worry keeps you from living large.

So why do we do it? Because we don't know any better. It's what we've been taught. It's all we know. It's how we react. It's why we're stuck. Now that you know that deep breathing is so tremendously healing, and worry is so detrimental, let's turn hope into action. Right here! Right now! We're going to take three deep breaths to reset our central nervous system. Breathe in through your nose and out through your mouth. Let's do that again—in and out. One last time, breathe in and out. Don't you feel better already? I'll tell you why. You feel better because when you breathe in deeply, you bring in new positive energy. When you breathe out through your mouth, you release old negative energy. So, there you have it!

Now I would like for you to pick one thing that you worry about every single day. It could be your health. It could be about your finances. It could be about your relationships, your happiness, or your mood. Now I want you to repeat these phrases, while you 'Tap' on the side of your wrist: Even though I have this worry about (just fill in the blank), I accept how I feel and forgive myself, even though I've been taught to worry. I accept who I am and forgive myself, even though I'm not sure how to change these old programs. I accept who I am and forgive myself. All this worry is stuck in my head. All this worry clouds my judgment. All this worry makes me panic. All this worry makes me stuck. All this worry makes me sick. All this worry, is it worth it? All this worry, why can't I release it? All this worry is so heavy to carry. All this worry has just become a bad habit. I'm ready to release this worry, these old programs, bad habits, and false beliefs from my mind, body, soul, and spirit right now.

Take a deep breath in and out. Release any and all thoughts, emotions, events, or memories not serving you right now.

My hope is that as you continue your quest for healing, you will take action! I place my faith in you to apply these healing insights to every aspect of your life, so you can have health, wealth, love, and happiness!

Healing Insight 59: "Yoga is delicious!"

YouTube Yoga Video

I must have picked up this little phrase along the way from one of the many YouTube videos that I watch daily. I tried to go back and find out what wonderful person said this so I could give them credit, but I still have not been able to find that one video. I'm going to give credit anyway to this wonderful person who was motivating me in more ways than one. Thank you!

I didn't realize how to apply this healing insight at first. I took it quite literally. I just figured yoga is good for you, so it makes sense that 'yoga is delicious!' Even though I love yoga so much I know that my body is not as flexible as I would like it to be. It doesn't do exactly what it should for the poses. In the beginning, it was a bit discouraging when I would look at the yoga instructor in the video because my body was doing something totally different. But I thought what the heck. I haven't been doing yoga for 20 years. I have many medical conditions. All I really need is some pain relief and flexibility. I don't need my body to do or look like that anyway.

Of course, with the lack of flexibility and muscle tone, yoga was a challenge for me and to be honest still is. Also, it was often uncomfortable. I would say to myself, "Yoga is delicious," during the most challenging times but once I learned how the body and the brain work, that they can be tricked to help you create healthy lifestyle habits, I knew how to use this healing insight. I knew that I could influence my brain to believe what I wanted it to. I continued to repeat this phrase every time I did yoga.

I knew that I was creating the plan with my conscious mind by saying, "Yoga is delicious!" I knew that my subconscious mind would carry out the plan so that I would be able to handle the yoga poses. That is the positive action I wanted to create to make yoga a healthy habit in my daily life.

This little phrase served two purposes. It encouraged me when I was being pushed to my limit. It also helped me to create a healthy lifestyle habit. I could see how this encouraging phrase was attracting positivity back to me! I felt excited that I was able to do yoga! As I repeated the phrase, it was helping me to repeat the action which was helping me to create the healthy habit. I caught on to this cycle because this was helping me to keep yoga as a daily routine.

So, I started applying 'is delicious' to many other things in my life. I have purchased many medical devices to help decrease pain or maintain relief. These medical devices are not always comfortable to use. My massage chair is fantastic but not when my trigger points were highly sensitive, I would say, "This massage is delicious!" My neck traction device is not always relaxing especially when my neck is super tight, and it is stretching it to its limit. Again, I would say, "This traction device is delicious!" My inversion table is the same way. It works wonders for my lower body and sciatic pain. But it's not always so great when you first get on. As always I would say to myself, "This is delicious," no matter what. The same goes for my TENS unit. It can give great relief. But at times it can be so strong or have the side effect of sensitivity to my skin. Of course, my TENS unit is 'just as delicious' as the other devices that I use.

I encourage you to find a phrase. Or use this one to keep you motivated. To help you trick your mind and your body to achieve a healthy lifestyle. This healing insight may seem silly but once you understand how it works—how the mind and body work; how the Law of Attraction works; how you can change your mind; how you can create healthy habits; how you can improve your life; how you can improve your health—you will believe this healing insight has great meaning.

I hope you are starting to understand how each of these concepts can be applied to your life. How these healing insights give you an explanation of how and why they work. How and why you must implement them into your life! I want to help you gain the full understanding of this information so you can feel the hope, the healing, and the peace. I want you to be successful in healing your mind, body, soul, and spirit! The main purpose of my course is to teach you how to use these healing insights to live your full life!

Healing Insight 60: The chains of habit are too light to be felt until they are too heavy to be broken.

Tai Lopez, *67 Steps*

Warren Buffet's powerful quote was shared by Tai Lopez, in his *67 Steps*. We all know that bad habits get the best of us. But what we didn't realize is that most of our everyday life is just a bad habit. This is because 95% of our day is run by our subconscious mind. So, these bad habits or 'programs' are just being repeated every single day! We don't even have to think about a bad habit; it just happens.

In his book, *The Power of Habit,* Charles Duhigg explains, "There are three parts to a habit, known as the habit loop. A cue is a trigger that tells your brain to automatically run the routine. The routine is a behavior (physical, mental, or emotional) that follows the cue. The reward is a positive incentive that tells your brain the routine is working great, so it is worth keeping." This allows the subconscious mind to run our programs. Remember, your brain and body are always looking for ways to be efficient to save time and energy! Also, the brain does not know the difference between a good or a bad habit.

But the author gives encouragement! If you can observe what the cue and reward are, you can change the routine! But you must be conscious! A technique called awareness training, which is used in the Alcoholics Anonymous Program, consists of having people describe why they do what they do. In other words, what cues or triggers their habitual behavior. This is the first step if you want to reverse a habit. Another interesting concept that AA requires is that people must attend 90 meetings in 90 days. Remember repetition is one of the four ways you can change your programs, according to Dr. Bruce Lipton. Also, it takes 66 days on average for people to acquire a new habit, according to the research study at University College London.

Now that you know how the brain and body work, that it takes repetition to change a habit, this will help you understand why you have so many bad habits because you have been repeating them; over and over and over for most of your life. It's not until you try to break a habit that you realize just how strong it really is. You grasp just how difficult it is to change or stop those bad habits that are haunting you every day.

Use this knowledge and turn your life around starting one habit at a time! You can wipe out old bad habits and replace them with new healthy habits. You can trick your mind with little phrases to send out that positive energy to attract it back to you. You can take action to show your brain and body that you are in control; you are conscious. You can give the conscious mind the plan (blueprint) that it needs. So the subconscious mind can carry out the plan to your benefit.

At Healing Insight 60, you must take responsibility for your own well-being! You have been through many of the healing insights. The process of how the brain and the body work and how the Law of Attraction works has been explained. You have also learned how consistent positive energy along with gratitude can propel your ability to accomplish anything! Now, it's time for you to realize that you must take action! You need to see the dirt. You need to create a plan. You need to write your goals on paper. You need to start reading those goals every day so that you can start sending out that positive energy so that you can allow the universe to work for your healing!

I hope at this point, in this book, you are not feeling like this is out of your reach because it's not! It's just knowledge, heck even common sense that you didn't know how to apply to your life. I want to help you realize what your BS story is. I want to help you understand the steps to change that BS story that's holding you back. I want to help you implement my proven 5-Step Process into your daily life! I want to guide you through this process to gently nurture your mind, body, soul, and spirit. To prime it for the healing that is about to take place! I want to partner with you to make this happen. Feel the hope, the healing, and the peace! So you can set this positive energy in motion!

Activity:

"On Cue!"

- List the cue, routine, and reward for one habit you want to change.

- List how long you have had this habit.

"On Cue!" Activity Sheet

Habit	
Cue	
Routine	
Reward	
How Long?	

Daily Challenge:

Turn Hope into Action!

"Get Physical!"

- Add the exercise/physical activity to your routine today!

- Commit to this healthy habit for at least 66 days!

- Make your new routine "Smoothielicious!"

- Try this Cherry Berry Smoothie Recipe!

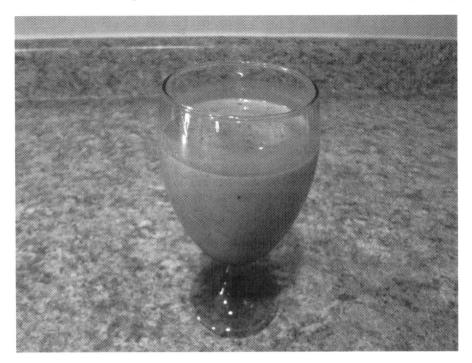

Cherry berry smoothie.

*Note: If possible shop for items that are organic, unsweetened, and do not contain preservatives.

- 1 Cup Coconut Water

- ½ Cup Frozen Cherries

- ½ Cup Frozen Blackberries

- 1 Frozen Banana

- 1 Tablespoon Cashew Butter

- 1 Tablespoon Chia Meal

Directions:

- Add all ingredients into blender or food processor.

- Blend well!

Enjoy!

Healing Insight 61: "I like to help people who help themselves."

Sheri Streeter, LMT, Massage by Sheri

This healing insight came to me before I could fully grasp its importance. Ms. Sheri was heaven sent. It felt like it was perfect timing when my primary physician referred me to her. I had asked him a handful of times for a referral to a massage therapist. The two massage therapists that he gave me referrals to are his personal providers. I believe that is the main reason he was so cautious before he mentioned my desire to them and shared their names with me. I was ecstatic that day! I said, "Score, now I can get a real massage!"

On my first visit with Ms. Sheri, I was scheduled for an hour session. She provides service out of her home. My GPS lost signal within a mile of her house. So, I called to let her know and to have her navigate me. I was a bit late, but she was understanding. I got so much more than a massage that day. I was given full attention. I felt like my concerns and experiences were completely acknowledged by her. She also had many of the same medical conditions and experiences as I did. We instantly connected. She mentioned to me that she had made it clear to my primary physician that she likes to help people who help themselves because it is hard work to help yourself feel better.

I didn't realize the level of service that she provided. Wow! She gave me so much in that one session alone. She demonstrated how to stretch my quads, my neck, and my shoulders. She showed me what equipment to use for deep pressure massage. She also had me try each stretch and use the equipment to be sure I was doing each one correctly. She told me where I could purchase the equipment as well as the price because she was so thorough. The session went over by a half hour. I apologized again for being late, but she assured me that it was fine because she wanted to give me what I needed to help relieve my pain.

She also suggested that I get a deep tissue massage and then follow up with a chiropractic adjustment to get the most benefit. She explained that because the bones and muscles are attached, they affect one another. I was so appreciative for all that she did for me. I bought the equipment she suggested immediately! I even bought one for my primary physician as a thank-you gift for all he had helped me with. I just wanted to spread the goodness!

I felt encouraged because she could see that I was already helping myself. Again, those intangibles were shining through. I think she was willing to share her suggestions with me because she was confident that I would follow through. She knew I was serious about wanting to help myself feel better. It was so much easier for me to add these new stretches to my routine. Not only because she showed me exactly what to do but also because she believed in me!

I want to help you find those intangibles that are inside of you. These intangibles will help you to create a space to heal. I want to be that inspiration for you! I want to be the motivation for you as well! I want you to know that I believe in you! I want you to know that I know your pain. I feel your pain. I know that you can help yourself! You can heal! You can live your full life!

Healing Insight 62: Have you reached max recovery?

Paul Kempton, MPT ATC, Kempton & Nelson Physical Therapy

This healing insight helped me realize that I was not going to settle for the physical status after two rounds of physical therapy treatment due to injuries from the car accident that I was involved in, in April of 2014. I had cervical sprain (whiplash) and a shoulder injury that was consistent with a rotator cuff injury. That day at therapy my usual provider was not available. So, I was treated by the lead physical therapist (the owner). At the end of the session, he asked me, "Do you feel like you have reached maximum recovery?" I hesitated to answer him. He went on to tell me that he had been involved in a car accident three years prior. He mentioned that he still had numbness in one of his legs. He also reminded me that after an injury we do not always recover 100%.

I told him that I understood that, but I had great benefits from dry needle therapy for TMJ. I had inquired with my regular physical therapist if that was a service that was provided at this physical therapy office. Since it was not, I had already talked with my doctor about getting a referral to the physical therapist who had treated me for TMJ. I explained this to the lead physical therapist and told him that yes, I believed I was ready to move on from the treatment at his facility, but that I still had hope that I could progress a bit more.

I share this healing insight with you for two reasons, number one because you know your body better than anyone else. Number two, because you must believe in yourself! You must believe that you can heal! I knew this even before I had the knowledge of how the body and brain work. How the Law of Attraction works. How maintaining a consistent attitude of gratitude will attract more positivity into your life. Dr. Joe Dispenza captures the essence of this belief in his quote, "The ultimate belief is the belief in yourself and in the field of infinite possibilities!"

I did transfer to the other physical therapist, and I received therapy for another two rounds. I did progress some. But my physical therapist helped me realize that there was something else holding me back from full recovery. That is why this book includes steps and techniques to heal your mind, body, soul, and spirit. Because of the mind, body, soul, and spirit connection, we need to understand what is holding us back. How to release it. How to move on. How to prime your central nervous system to heal.

I want to help you realize that you must heal at every level! I want to help you know the steps of how to accomplish that! I want to help you understand how you can create a space to heal! I want to give you everything you need to succeed! Fibromyalgia and many other medical conditions that we deal with are difficult to live with on a day-to-day basis. That's why I'm sharing this insight, so that you can wrap your mind around them all and take action to find relief today!

Healing Insight 63: You don't have to be symptomatic.

Blaine Brooks, PT, DPT, Kinect Physical Therapy

This healing insight was probably the most important insight of them all! Blaine Brooks, my awesome physical therapist, is responsible for this healing insight. He also guided me on how to journal what I was feeling in my daily symptom log, while I was being treated for TMJ. But sometimes, I am so mule-headed, or maybe I was just so stuck in the stress response cycle, that I pretty much had to have this insight spelled out for me.

I was on my second round of physical therapy for the car accident injuries. My therapist was so good at picking apart my symptoms and figuring out what was aggravating my injuries. But after a while I had him stumped or maybe just frustrated. He told me straight out, "You know you can have an injury without being symptomatic." I thought about this. I didn't even respond that I can remember. He went on to explain that our pain is not always physical.

He said, "So, if your pain is not physical, then what are you holding onto?" I really didn't know how to respond. I was in the hot seat! I didn't really feel embarrassed. I was just speechless because it had never crossed my mind. I knew about psychosomatic symptoms. I was taught this term while earning my degree as an OT assistant. But it never crossed my mind that this might be what was going on with me. Once again, my education had gone out the window.

My therapist was aware that I had been using Emotional Freedom Techniques (EFT) Tapping Meditation to help me work through my many medical conditions. I would bring him up to date as I realized that I was making some progress. I had mentioned to him in so many words that I didn't have much of a relationship with my mother. We had discussed here and there the loss of my family members. He knew that my finances were strained.

My answer was right in front of my face. These situations were the dirt that I hadn't been willing to see. These situations were my BS story that was holding me back. It was all those emotions that I had kept bottled up and forced down my entire life. This was how that consistent attitude focused on anger had become my personality. The emotions related to these situations were making me sick! I was so grateful for Blaine's awareness and honesty.

There's only one other time that I can remember in my life that a good friend of mine was straightforward with me when I needed it the most. She told me, I had to stop feeling sorry for myself after my father passed away. So once again, here I was faced with the reality that I needed to get off the pity pot. I needed to start helping myself process and release these emotions, memories, and events causing me emotional, physical, and spiritual pain.

But there was an enormous difference this time. I was immersed in all this self-development. I was learning how my mind and body worked. I knew I was no longer a victim of my genetics. I was no longer a victim of a scarcity mindset. I used Tapping Meditation with this healing insight specifically. Every time my neck or my shoulder hurt I said to myself, "I can have an injury without being symptomatic." I would repeat, "You don't have to be symptomatic."

I had three more therapy sessions left that were allowed for my insurance in February of 2017 but when my insurance changed it wouldn't be effective until April 2017. So, I would have to wait to finish those last three sessions. I seriously considered finishing the last three sessions. I even called the therapy office to find out if I could still resume my therapy with Blaine. I was assured that I could resume whenever my insurance was active again. I told the therapist that I would phone back once my insurance was effective.

During that time frame, I was using Tapping Meditation with this insight. I also kept doing my physical therapy home program daily. Every time I hurt I just told myself, "You don't have to be symptomatic." By the time my insurance became effective, I decided that I was okay. I didn't need to resume my physical therapy. Because I could have an injury and I didn't have to be symptomatic.

I share this healing insight with you because I want to stress how significant the connection between the body, mind, soul, and spirit really is. I also want to stress how important it is to process and release emotions, memories, and thoughts that are holding you back. Another crucial factor involved in the healing insight is you must see the dirt before you can clean it up! I hope that you will take action! I want to help you learn how to take responsibility for your own well-being! I want to help you realize that your thoughts matter! You matter!

Healing Insight 64: The brain believes what it is repeatedly told.

All Thought Leaders

I originally wanted this healing insight to be, "Your symptoms are consistent with a 60-year-old!" But I was sure it wouldn't seem like much of a healing insight. As I mentioned in Healing Insight 8, I would wake up and the first thought in my mind was, *oh f*** my life sucks, I feel like a 90-year-old woman, my life is a joke, I just want to be dead!* So, when my awesome physical therapist told me that my symptoms were consistent with a 60-year-old woman, I took his comment as a compliment. I saw it as proof that the Law of Attraction was working!

I had changed my inner dialogue every morning when I woke up. I started telling myself, "I feel amazing!" even before I got out of bed. "I love my life. My body feels great. I can't wait to live this brand-new, never-lived-in day!" So, his comment was the evidence that I had I shaved off 30 years from feeling like a 90-year-old woman. Now I was only displaying symptoms of a 60-year-old woman. Hallelujah! You're probably thinking that I'm crazy, but that's okay because this helped me fuel my positive energy. It helped fuel my energy so much that I rushed home to tell my family the good news.

I kept repeating this new dialogue to myself every morning. Every time I had pain in my shoulder or neck, I said, "I don't have to be symptomatic just because I have an injury." The week after, I went to see my neurologist. When he looked at my chart, he glanced up at me and said, "Forty-five? You look like you're only thirty-five." I just smiled and said, "Oh I wish I was thirty-five again." I thought to myself, well, I just shaved off another 25 years. Wow! This stuff really does work! Of course, when I shared this with my family they laughed. But again, it powered my positive energy.

I discussed with my family at what age I would have to be to reverse back all the way to where I would be pain-free. When I figured it out, I would have to shave off another ten years. I realized that I had been in chronic pain since I was 26 years old. I lost my father when I was 23 years old. As I mentioned before, this was the first and the most devastating loss that I have experienced in my life. So, when I look back now, it does not surprise me that by age 26 I was in chronic pain.

The events that took place around the time of my father's illness the month that he was in the hospital, plus the events that followed his death around his funeral arrangements, just piled up. I didn't know how to process and release them, so I just stuffed them down. That's when the chronic pain was triggered. Then all the other life events occurred. The financial burdens, the loss of more family members, and more stress around the relationship with my mother. The emotions, thoughts, and memories that weren't serving me were just compounded until finally, my body couldn't handle it anymore.

I hope you can see the connection between mind, body, soul, and spirit in both my life and yours. I want to help you be able to stop the negative cycle of energy that you are stuck in. I want to help you realize how you can apply these healing insights to every aspect of your life. I want to help you break free from being in the stress response cycle that is causing the imbalance in your energy system. Look at what's been going on in your life. Examine what thoughts, emotions, and memories you are holding on to. Find the courage, use your inner strength, and decide to take back your health, take control of your life, and find relief today!

Healing Insight 65: You can exercise your core every day.

Blaine Brooks, PT, DPT, Kinect Physical Therapy

Another wonderful healing insight from the exceptional physical therapist that helped me realize I did not have to be symptomatic. I must have picked up this information somewhere during my studies to become an occupational therapy assistant. But once again, I was unable to access or apply this information to my situation due to being in a stress response cycle. This healing insight was important because my core has been such a source of pain, excruciating pain. I knew that I needed to strengthen my core more than anything. I had a 12-inch incision to remove my left ovary that hemorrhaged in 2003. This surgery damaged my muscle tissue and made my core muscles very weak.

A little bonus insight, pain occurs because of two reasons. When muscles are weak and when muscles are overused. That is why this healing insight was so crucial for me. If I planned on reducing or preventing pain in my core muscles, pelvic area, and bladder, I needed to strengthen my core. This healing insight was heaven sent. It meant that I had a chance to build some muscle in my core to help reduce pain. Of course, I took this information and ran with it.

I figured out ways to do core strength exercises throughout my daily routine. I made sure that my yoga routine included planks, leg lifts, and other core strength exercises. Even while I was waiting at the doctor's or watching a movie at the theater, I did core exercises by just lifting my feet off the floor one at a time. This healing insight is more valuable than you might first think, because fibromyalgia has so many other related medical conditions that affect the pelvic area and the core muscles.

Fibromyalgia causes you to be so fatigued. It drains every ounce of your energy out of you every single day of your life. This causes you to either sit still or lie down because you want to minimize your pain and rest as much as you can. But remember, every second that you rest, sleep, or lie down you're not using any of your muscles. Your core muscles are the center of your stability. Your core muscles are the muscles that help you sit, stand, move around in bed, and walk. So please do not take this healing insight lightly.

This applies to all of your muscles. When you are not using your muscles, they waste away. The medical term is called atrophy. I knew this information from my educational background. But it didn't matter because all I could think of was the pain. I just wanted relief. I thought if I didn't move then the pain would go away. I thought if I took my prescription medications the pain would go away. I thought I would feel better, but I didn't. All that happened was that I was drugged up asleep on my couch. When I woke up, I was in pain again. So, I took more pills, got drugged up, fell asleep on the couch, once again, and the cycle continued.

Please take this healing insight for its full value. Realize that you can exercise your core every day. It is your core that supports every part of your daily life. The core is a great place to start strengthening your muscles. To help you reduce pain from the many medical conditions related to fibromyalgia. I hope this healing insight will give you some basic knowledge, as well as motivation and useful ideas so you can start improving your health.

As you can see, I didn't start my physical activity routine with much. I didn't increase the number of minutes either. I just found time throughout my day to add in as many yoga routines, exercise routines, and stretch routines as I could. I think people get trapped thinking they need to dedicate a whole hour to a workout routine. That is not realistic or even possible with the diagnosis of fibromyalgia. Realize that five minutes is plenty. Even one minute will give you relief if that's where you need to start.

Whether you have a medical diagnosis or not, The 5-Step Process can be applied to all areas of your life! These five steps are the foundation for using these healing insights daily! You matter! You are worthy of having the steps you need to create the life you deserve! My plan is to help you realize that you can maximize for a full life, then give you the tools you need to succeed!

Healing Insight 66: Actually, it is that simple.

Bleed for This, based on the true story of Vinny Pazienza, Ben Younger

As you have seen in Healing Insight 39, "War Room Journal," these healing insights can come from anywhere, even a movie. The true story of Vinny Pazienza, in the movie *Bleed for This,* touched my heart so deeply. Vinny's spirit, will, fight, and ability to think positive thoughts are what helped him to heal again. He was able to take action. He sent out the message that was so in sync that he was able to attract his health back to him, get his life back, and find relief.

He showed how consistent self-care was the foundation to start healing. Because he was an amazing athlete, he understood that repetition was the key. He knew that by taking action, he could start this powerful healing ability in himself. In one interview he said, "Actually, it is that simple." That sentence made me realize that yes, it is! I can't stress how important that factor is. I'm sure I've said it more times than you want to hear in this book, but you must take action!

You cannot continue to allow your subconscious mind to run those old programs, false beliefs, and bad habits that are holding you back. If you want to take control of your life and find relief today, then you must stop this cycle of negative energy! Proof that the Law of Attraction works is right in front of your eyes. Take a good look at my life. Look at your life! Look around you. Do you see it? Remember the concept of the Law of Attraction is 'like attracts like.'

Actually, it is that simple. If you think negative you get negative; if you think positive, you get positive results. I'm going to say it again. It's that simple! Please understand that I'm not being sarcastic. I push you only because I know where you are right now. I push you because damn it, you are worth it! You are worthy just by being born. It's okay if you didn't value you own self-worth before because I'm here to show you that you are worth it.

So, use me as a tool, a resource, support, a mentor. Learn from my life. Learn from my mistakes. You don't have to learn the hard way! That's a false belief. You can look at other people's lives and reverse-engineer your life. That simply means look at what you're doing. Look what others are doing. Figure out what isn't working. Then remove what isn't working and put in what does work. It is that simple!

I want to help you to do this because I know you're worth it! Accept my help and kickstart your healing today! You have these healing insights. You understand these concepts. You have the blueprint for success. Now take action! Apply this knowledge to your own life! Free yourself from those strong chains of habit that are holding you back! Dig deep, find that fire that still exists inside you! It's okay if your flame is burning low. Because now you know how to take back your energy. Elevate it to its full potential!

Now you know that you can invite abundance into your life. Now you know how to send out those abundant invitations to the universe. So, what are you waiting for? Remember, change must take place for you to create a space to heal! Action must take place for you to make change! You must have feelings that are on the same wavelength as your thoughts before you can take action! Positive thoughts must take place before your feelings can match them! So, it is that simple! Start this cycle of positive energy in your life by having a positive thought. You must maximize for a full life today! Today is the only day that is guaranteed. The past cannot be changed. The future may never be. You must make that change today!

Healing Insight 67: Keep doing what you're doing.

Dr. Fairfax, AZ ArthroCare

This healing insight made me realize I must be doing something right. I have been under a rheumatologist's care since 2013. Early on Dr. Fairfax prescribed some different fibromyalgia pain medication. At the time, I had elevated liver enzyme levels, so I didn't try all of them. The ones I did try seemed to have more side effects than benefits. I mentioned to him throughout my treatment that I was doing Tapping Meditation and yoga daily.

During one visit, he asked me how long I was able to do yoga. I told him it depended on my energy level. But it could be anywhere from five to twenty minutes. He was still impressed with the fact that I even did yoga. When my liver enzyme levels became normal, I was not willing to add any new medications to my treatment. I feared that my liver enzymes levels would be elevated again. Plus, I was so far into this healing journey that I didn't want to contaminate my body with any more toxins.

Dr. Fairfax was okay with me not trying any more medications because he respected my decision. I had already stopped taking pregabalin with the guidance of my primary physician in June of 2016. So, by the time I went to see my rheumatologist in December of 2016, I had a good handle on my symptoms. I had remembered what my primary physician said when I was trying to stop my heartburn medications. He suggested preventing symptoms from happening rather than soothing them after the fact. I took that healing insight and I applied it to every symptom that I had.

I designed my day to include routines to prevent my symptoms from happening, if possible. For instance, I would 'Tap,' meditate, stretch, or exercise in bed before I got up. While I was brushing my teeth, I would do a hip rotation routine. While I was eating breakfast, I would do a hip stretch routine and apply an ice pack to whatever body part might need attention that day. I used my donut-shaped cushion to relieve perineal discomfort throughout the day. I changed positions every thirty minutes to alleviate any discomfort or pain.

I would take five-minute stretch or yoga breaks. I did my physical therapy home program which included exercise and stretches for my jaw, neck, shoulders, hips, and sacroiliac joint. I kept a low acidic diet to reduce or eliminate my bladder symptoms. I continued to eat healthily. I kept taking my vitamins and supplements. Many of them were part of the 10-Day Detox Diet that I started in 2014. I would use my medical equipment to keep my symptoms to a minimum.

So, when Dr. Fairfax discharged me from his care, I realized how much I was helping myself daily. He said, "You can follow up with me if you feel it's necessary. I'm not prescribing or monitoring you for any medication. Just keep doing what you're doing." At first, I thought oh no. But then I figured, I got this! I have learned so much from these healing insights. I had changed my thoughts, feelings, as well as processed and released so much of what was not serving me. I had taken action! I had attracted positive energy back into my life! I had created a space to heal! I had chosen to take responsibility for my own well-being! I had learned how self-care and nurturing my body, mind, soul, and spirit could help me create a pain-free life and love every minute of it!

I don't know if I had realized how much progress I had made until that day. I was so busy trying to feel better. I didn't realize I was feeling better! I was just focused on keeping my pain and symptoms minimal. If possible, I was keeping my symptoms from bothering me at all. I had applied these healing insights to my life.

Little by little these healing insights were added to my daily life. Now I understood how to create a healthy lifestyle. As I think back I am amazed because I didn't realize healing my mind, body, soul, and spirit was possible. I had been in such a cycle of unhealthy living, it seemed like I was climbing Mount Everest most of the time. I want to point out that consistency, repetition, and a steady attitude of gratitude is what will help you take action to create the life you deserve!

Healing Insight 68: The more you exercise, the stronger you get; the less pain you have!

Dr. Castellanos, Dignity Health Medical Group-Pelvic Pain Clinic

Another super simple healing insight, this time from my gynecologist. This is another provider that I wondered if I had met by chance. But with all my understanding of how the Law of Attraction works, I know this was meant to be. I was blessed to be referred to Dr. Castellanos at the Pelvic Pain Clinic by the wonderful allergist physician's assistant that got me started on this journey in the first place. She had mentioned that she too had visited the Pelvic Pain Clinic. She shared some of the treatment options they had available. She was still not sure that their services would be something that would benefit her. But that didn't stop her from giving me their contact information, so I could find out for myself.

I felt the same way the day I drove to my first appointment at the Pelvic Pain Clinic as I did the day that I met her. All the same thoughts came up. I wasn't up to starting from scratch with a new provider. But I knew that the other provider I had was not a good fit. I was still having pain in my bladder and my pelvic area. It still felt like I had a match burning in my genital area. That must have been what made me keep the appointment that day. I did end up needing another pelvic surgery which I mentioned that I had done in January of 2015. But finding the services of this facility was another piece to the puzzle that I needed to discover on this healing journey.

I never felt so validated. Dr. Castellanos is a wonderful listener much like my primary physician. He doesn't make me feel like my pain is not real. He doesn't make me feel like I don't understand my own body. He doesn't make me feel like I must prove to him that my symptoms are intense. He not only listens but offers treatment options with no pressure. He always makes me feel like he has plenty of time.

He was very pleased with my report of less pain in March 2017. I explained to him that I was doing my pelvic floor physical therapy home program daily. I also mentioned that I was still using Tapping Meditation. I was practicing yoga. I was keeping a low-acid diet for my bladder. He simply said, "The more you exercise, the stronger you get; the less pain you have." I knew this, but somehow it just felt good to hear it from someone else.

It was more proof that what I was doing was working! It showed me that I had made such strong connections that I had created new healthy lifestyle habits. Dr. Joe Dispenza refers to these connections as 'neural nets.' It made me realize that I was doing a much better job of nurturing my mind, body, soul, and spirit. It made me appreciate my new belief in functional medicine. To remind you, functional medicine is treating the cause, not the symptoms, through the process of taking responsibility for your own self-care.

The self-care I was providing consistently to every level of my being was exactly what I needed. Again, it was nice to get this feedback from someone other than myself or a family member. It made it so much more valuable. I've never been one to sugarcoat anything. So maybe that's why this healing insight was so powerful. I reminded Dr. Castellanos at the end of my appointment to please share the information that I had given him about TheTappingSolution.com. He was also excited to hear about how my primary physician and I had come up with a little trick to create a homemade vaginal suppository. He said he would pass that on to his patients as well.

It's so comforting and exhilarating at the same time to know that I have such a wonderful medical team! It is amazing how much I have learned from each of them. But it is also satisfying that I can contribute. Not only to my own health care, but to the health care of others. In this sensitive, painful situation, I am pleased that my providers are willing to listen as well as share information that they feel is valuable to other patients.

My hope in sharing this healing insight is that you can understand that what you do matters! What you think matters! What you feel matters! Your actions matter! Your attitude matters! Your beliefs matter! Your programs matter! You matter! I want to help you understand how daily nurturing self-care along with these healing insights can help you find pain relief today!

I want to help you understand fully how you can take responsibility for your own well-being. To find those intangibles that are inside of you. That you have always had and that are just waiting to shine through. Those intangibles will push you to perform at your highest ability. I want to motivate you to take action so that you can have a pain-free life and love every minute of it!

Healing Insight 69: Use it or lose it!

Breaking the Habit of Being Yourself: How to Lose Your Mind and Create a New One, Dr. Joe Dispenza

This healing insight is one that I'm sure most everyone has heard. It applies to most everything in life. This concept is simple. If you don't use it, you lose it. Dr. Joe Dispenza explains it like this: "Nerve cells that no longer fire together, no longer wire together. This is the universal law of 'use it or lose it' in action, and it can work wonders in changing old paradigms of thought about ourselves."

This concept can be used for you as well as against you. Let's relate this to a bad habit. If you keep having the same thoughts, emotions, and actions, your body releases the same hormones. This process strengthens that connection. So, the bad habit will be stronger and harder to break.

You can also use it to get rid of bad habits. Remember, if you don't use it, you lose it. So, it's that simple. Just don't use it and then you will lose it. If you interrupt your thoughts, you change your emotions, mindset, programs, false beliefs, and attitude. Then you are not running your old programs. So, your old programs will fade because you are not using those connections. Eventually, your old programs, false beliefs, thoughts, feelings, actions, reactions, and old habits will disappear. It's like magic!

You can also use this healing insight to your advantage to create a new habit. One way to reprogram the brain is through repetition, repetition, repetition. This repetition will make the connection stronger and stronger and stronger. Then you will end up with an awesome healthy habit. Again, another simple concept with tremendous healing insight! Now I urge you to start using it. Start making those connections to new programs, new beliefs, and new healthy habits!

I hope that I can help you! To motivate you so you can start creating a new mindset, new programs, new beliefs, and new healthy habits. I offer my help, my hand to support you. I want to show you how simple this process truly is. It may not be easy in the beginning. But you can use these healing insights to your advantage to fool your body and your mind. To let go of things that are not serving you. To build strong, healthy connections that will give you lasting change. The hard work is worth it!

Remember, I was in your shoes. In pain constantly, around the clock. Hurting, suffering, and torturing myself. I was searching. I was scrambling. I was desperate to find the answer for pain relief! I wanted my health back! I wanted control of my life! The support I offer can give you what you need to get your health back, to get control of your life and to find relief today, just like I did. This is possible! I have laid out exactly how to do it! I hope you will allow me to give you the support that I know you will need on your quest to heal.

There is no reason why you can't create a space to heal! There's no reason why you can't help yourself! There is no reason why you can't heal yourself! I hope this healing insight will serve as proof that these possibilities are available to you. That you can make the changes you need to make in your body, and in your life. I hope that by sharing my story, you can realize you are worth it! Understand that there is hope, healing, and peace!

Even though this message was not clear or taught to you before, I am grateful that I can share these healing insights with you now. I would have never imagined that my journey through hell would eventually lead me to the understanding of how I could create 'heaven on Earth.' Iyanla Vanzant is so wise, she says, "Everything is and was just as it needs to be." She's right! Recognize that your situation, no matter how difficult it is right now, can and will get better! You can achieve health, wealth, love, and happiness!

Healing Insight 70: Chanting heals!

Deborah Lucero

This healing insight is what allowed me to finally stop the pelvic floor spasms after two and half weeks. I was still a bit weary after meditating because the spasms did not stop immediately. Meditation alone had worked for me to stop taking my other muscle spasm medications. So, I thought I needed an extra boost. I Googled the mantra for the root chakra. I chanted the word 'Lam' for twenty minutes straight! That's what the mantra required to clear the root chakra. I felt all the higher-level emotions (safety, comfort, security, protection, love, forgiveness, self-love, self-forgiveness, humility, empowerment, gratitude, thankfulness, blessed, connected, whole, and unity with the universe) as I did this chanting.

When I was finished, I felt some relief. But my spasms were still there. I said to myself, "Oh crap, I already threw out my medications, so I can't fall back on those, what do I do now?" I still believed in this technique because it had worked for me before. But it had already been two and a half weeks of nonstop spasms. I needed some relief now! I said to myself, "If I don't feel better by noon today, I will call in to request a refill on my medications." I was hoping that's all I needed to do, and I wouldn't have to schedule an appointment. 12:00 rolled around and still I didn't want to call the doctor. About 12:30 my pain and my muscle spasms stopped and had not returned. I couldn't believe it! I knew it was possible! I had done it! I was so happy, amazed, grateful, and thankful! I felt every emotion in that moment of time. I said to myself, "I am the placebo!"

By Thursday of that week, I felt like I was having symptoms of a urinary tract infection (UTI). I thought, here we go again, this body is going to reject the fact that I am taking over. But I said, "My brain is going to be in control. My subconscious is not going to just run all day long. I am tired of being a zombie in pain." I meditated, this time using the Teyata Om mantra to rid my body of the UTI symptoms. This meditation is used to release negative energy and promote health. I felt those higher-level emotions, once more. I had some relief but not total relief.

My youngest son needed a ride at 1:00 that day to volunteer at the library. Again, my 'Western Medicine' mindset told me, "If you don't feel better by the time you drop him off at the library, stop by Urgent Care on the way home to do a urinalysis." But I didn't give up! I said, "If meditation along with feeling these higher-level emotions can work on muscle spasms, it can work on UTI symptoms too!" It did work again! I was overjoyed! I said, "Wow, look what I can do! I learned this! I figured it out! I made the connection between my thoughts my feelings match! I sent out that positive energy! I let the universe know that I felt it in every fiber of my being, at every level of consciousness!"

The importance of how your mind can make things happen may be difficult to realize. My whole focus of this book is to help you grasp all of this! To help you make this connection! To help you follow The 5-Step Process. To teach you how to master your ability to heal yourself! I want to show you how you can use these techniques to feel the hope, the healing, and the peace!

The best way for me to help you understand this is to have you think back to a time when everything seemed hopeless. But even though it felt that way, you still found something inside of you. That little flame that hadn't burned out. You fostered it. You nurtured it. You believed in it. You placed your hope and your faith in it. You felt it no matter what. You knew that something good would come from it. Remember how you felt, every emotion! Remember how you knew that everything would be okay! Remember how you were able to see the possibilities! Feel how you felt, at that moment! Apply those higher-level emotions to the fact that you want to heal. Apply those emotions to whatever symptom is bothering you, at this moment. Feel the gratitude right now as if what you desire has already happened!

Dr. Joe Dispenza explains it like this: "The emotional signature of gratitude means the event has already happened." If you can be grateful ahead a time for future blessings, you are telling the brain that the event has already happened. You can trick the brain because it believes what it is repeatedly told. Remember, the brain does not know the difference between past, present, or future. The brain will believe that your gratitude is sincere when your thoughts and your emotions match. It will send out positive energy through the emotional signature of gratitude to the universe to invite abundance into your life. By expressing gratitude, you will draw what you desire back to you!

So, you can create a space to heal! You can help yourself! You can heal yourself! You can live the life you deserve! You can live a pain-free life and love every minute of it! You can achieve health, wealth, love, and happiness! You can honor your mind, body, soul, and spirit! You can live your full life!

Activity:

"Restore Your Mind, Body, Soul & Spirit!" Restorative Yoga Chair Routine:

"We need these moments of stillness so that the body can heal."

~rachel@sleepysantosha.com~

How does restorative yoga work?

As with any form of yoga, RY uses specific poses, but it also makes use of various props to provide the utmost comfort to support and promote relaxation.

Each pose is linked to a specific system within your body.

Along with poses that alleviate head and back pains, there are even specific RY classes and poses designed for people suffering from cancer.

The goal of RY is to unlearn chronic stress and pain responses to give the mind or retrain the mind to healthier healing responses.

Relaxation specifically helps improve pain and reduces stress. Stress promotes pain and its occurrence.

Unlike other styles of yoga, in RY, the poses are meant to be held for 10 minutes or longer. This is to attain a complete state of relaxation and elicit the relaxation response with gentle yoga poses and conscious breathing.

Instructions:

Child's Pose (Arms Forward):

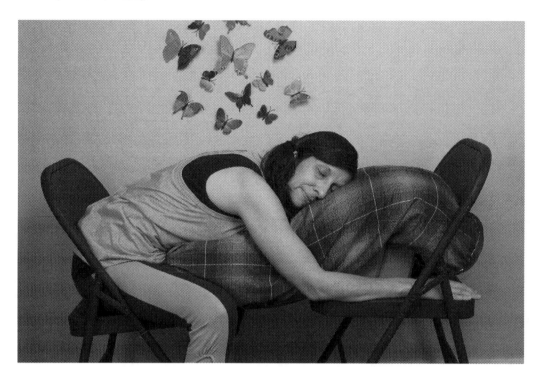

Child's pose (arms forward).

- Place 2 chairs facing each other.

- Place bolster at an incline with one end resting on the chair and the other end resting at the desired height on yoga block or books.

- Lean forward; rest your body and head on the bolster.

- Turn head to one side.

- Place hands on the chair in front of you.

- Hold the pose for 30 seconds to 10 minutes.

- Turn head to the other side and repeat.

Remember: The RY poses are meant to be held for up to 10 minutes.

Sleeping Pigeon Pose:

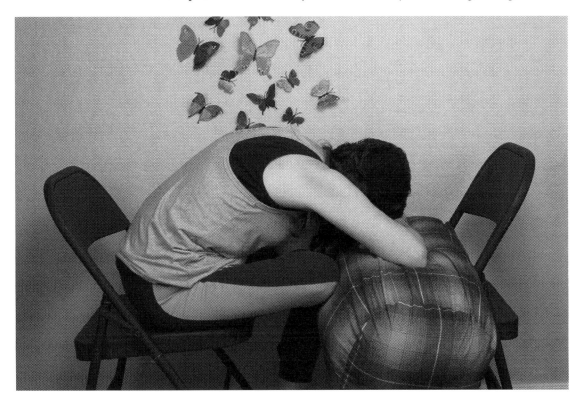

Sleeping pigeon pose.

- Place bolster across the chair in front of you.

- Place one foot on opposite knee.

- Lean forward.

- Rest head on the forearms.

- Hold the pose for 30 seconds to 10 minutes.

- Switch legs and repeat.

Remember: This pose would be held for up to 10 minutes as well, so you can achieve maximum relaxation!

Healing Points to Treasure

1. Realize that when you are in the stress response cycle, you do not think clearly! you cannot think clearly!

2. Taking deep breaths calms your central nervous system. It helps you access the part of your parasympathetic nervous system which controls healing!

3. The body and the brain can be tricked to help you create healthy lifestyle habits.

4. Most of your everyday life is just a bad habit. 95% of your day is run by your subconscious mind. So, bad habits or 'programs' are just being repeated every single day!

5. People are encouraged when they see you helping yourself. They are willing to share suggestions because they are confident that you will follow through!

6. You know your body better than anyone else. You must believe in yourself!

7. Realize what you are holding onto. Start helping yourself process and release emotions, memories, and events that are causing you emotional, physical, and spiritual pain.

8. Remember, the brain believes what it is repeatedly told! This is proof that the Law of Attraction works!

9. Pain occurs when muscles are weak and when muscles are overused. When you are not using your muscles, they waste away. The medical term is called atrophy.

10. Actually, it is that simple! If you think negative you get negative; if you think positive, you get positive results.

11. Prevent symptoms from happening rather than soothing them after the fact. Design your day to include routines to prevent symptoms from happening, if possible. 'Tap,' meditate, stretch, or exercise.

12. What you do matters! What you think matters! What you feel matters! Your actions matter! Your attitude matters! Your beliefs matter! Your programs matter! You matter!

13. Get rid of bad habits. Remember, if you don't use it, you lose it. Eventually, your old programs, false beliefs, thoughts, feelings, actions, reactions, and old habits will disappear. It's like magic!

14. The brain does not know the difference between past, present, or future. It will believe your gratitude is sincere when your thoughts and emotions match. By expressing gratitude, you will draw what you desire back to you! So, you can live your full life!

Healing Insights Summary

You can't wait for the mystical moment to feel awe, in fact, you have to feel awe for the mystical moment to occur. You have to feel love for a new relationship to show up, you have to feel empowered in order to have success, you have to feel wholeness before healing can occur.

(Dr. Joe Dispenza)

This quote by Dr. Dispenza clarifies how you can access the power of your subconscious mind. What a wonderful feeling. Just as you must feel the awe, you must understand how this magnificent power is fueled by a thought. Create a positive thought. No matter what you think, the Law of Attraction will return your thought to you as reality. I trust that you will master my proven 5-Step Process so you can maximize for a full life!

My desire is for you to turn hope into action! Believe in yourself and decide today to lead your life with an abundant mindset! My dream is society will be taught this healing wisdom as children. I never want anyone to feel as hopeless and helpless as I did! Once again, I urge you to turn these Healing Insights into healthy daily habits! Say yes to life! Live your full life! :)

These healing insights changed my life forever! I just had to take action. Once I did I realized how simple it was to BE F*#ING **AMAZING!** My book can change your life too! Master this knowledge. Apply it to your life and BE F*#ING **AMAZING!**

The 5-Step Process Cheat Sheet

"For life is about movement, movement of being."

~James Van Praagh~

It is by honoring your mind, body, soul, and spirit that you can access movement of being!

I have created a cheat sheet for you to follow The 5-Step Process.

Step 1 Detox: Detox your mind, body, soul, and spirit from thoughts, emotions, events, relationships, unhealthy food, old programs, false beliefs, and bad habits!

Step 2 Releasing Emotion: Use Emotional Freedom Techniques (Tapping Meditation) to access the process of super learning to push the record button on the subconscious mind to fully process and release what is not serving you!

Step 3 Mindset: Use an abundant mindset to free yourself from being in a chronic stress response cycle. Listen to what your body needs. Listen to your soul to know what emotions need to be processed and released from your mind. Listen to your spirit; to live your truth, your purpose, and realize your full potential!

Step 4 Reprogramming Your Mind: The secret to this process is basking in the emotions of gratitude ahead of time. Feel all those emotions that you usually do when you have received a blessing. Once you surrender completely you will attract what you sent out. Your thoughts will become a reality!

Step 5 Exercise/Physical Activity: Use movement to keep your energy centers (chakras) clear and moving freely. Find the little flame that hasn't burned out. Nurture it. Believe in it. Place your hope and your faith in it. Know that something good will come from it. See the possibilities!

I leave you with the definition of spirit.

"In spirit, you are connected; you are being your true self."

~James Van Praagh~

A Special Note

Are you ready to maximize for a full life? I have included this bonus section for everyone who Turned Hope into Action and finished the book. I commend you for taking responsibility for your personal well-being. Congratulations!

If you are still reading this, you are ready to live your full life! By taking action, you have shown me that you are committed to improving your health, life, and realizing your full potential. I hope that what you learned in this book will help you detox, release emotions not serving you, create a positive mindset, reprogram your mind, and add exercise and physical activity to your daily life.

If you are ready to start the process of healing your mind, body, soul, and spirit to create the life you deserve, I have something to kickstart your healing!

As a special gift for believing in yourself and taking the first step, please accept the Tapping Meditation for Forgiveness. You can access this gift at gift.liveyourfulllife.com. The Tapping Meditation script is absolutely free!

This special gift is for everyone who made it this far! So, please let others **"BE F*#%ING AMAZING"** just like you and earn access to this link!

Thank you!

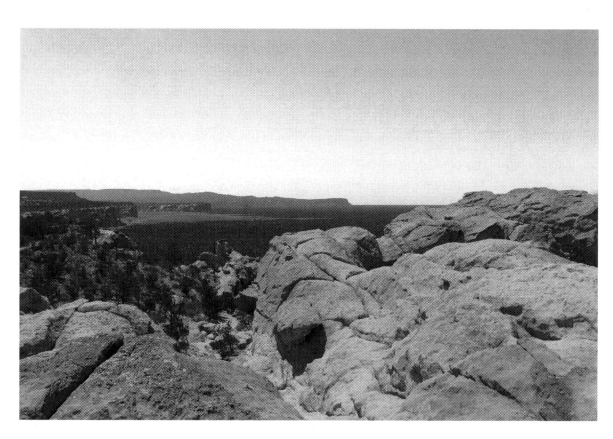

"Everyone knows how to choose; few know how to let go. But it's only by letting go of each experience that you make room for the next. The skill of letting go can be learned, and once learned you will enjoy living much more spontaneously."
~Deepak Chopra~

Resource—Newsletter List

* *The Blood Sugar Solution 10-Day Detox Diet*, Dr. Mark Hyman http://drhyman.com/

* *The Tapping Solution: A Revolutionary System for Stress-Free Living*, Nick Ortner http://www.nickortner.com/ https://www.thetappingsolution.com/

* *Awaken the Giant Within, MONEY Master the Game*, Tony Robbins https://www.tonyrobbins.com/

* Louse Hay, Hay House Publishing https://www.hayhouse.com/

* *The Placebo Effect, Biology of Belief, How to Live Heaven on Earth* (YouTube), Dr. Bruce Lipton https://www.brucelipton.com/

Overcoming the Past: Trauma, the Shadow, and the Inner Child, podcast compliments of Hay House Radio, Teal Swan https://tealswan.com/

* *Hay House U Live 2017 Conference*, James Van Praagh http://www.vanpraagh.com/

Power of Your Subconscious Mind, Dr. Joseph Murphy https://www.facebook.com/DrJosephMurphyTrust/

The 7 Habits of Highly Effective People, Stephen R. Covey https://www.stephencovey.com/

The Five Love Languages, Gary Chapman http://www.5lovelanguages.com/gary-chapman/

Functional Health Summit, Dr. Axe https://draxe.com/

"Surrogate" Tapping Meditation, Jessica Ortner http://www.jessicaortner.com/ https://www.thetappingsolution.com/

Truth About Cancer Summit 2015 https://thetruthaboutcancer.com/2015-the-truth-about-cancer-year-in-review/ Ard Pisa, Author, Researcher & Speaker https://www.facebook.com/ard.pisa

Quantum Enigma, Bruce Rosenblum and Fred Kuttner http://quantumenigma.com/about-the-authors/

67 Steps, Tai Lopez http://www.tailopez.com

The One Thing: The Surprisingly Simple Truth Behind Extraordinary Results, Gary Keller and Jay Papasan https://www.the1thing.com/

War Room: Prayer is a Powerful Weapon, from the creators of *Fireproof* and *Courageous* https://warroomthemovie.com/

The Magic of Thinking Big, David J. Schwartz https://en.wikipedia.org/wiki/David_J._Schwartz_(motivational_writer)

Annual Tapping World Summit, Carol Look, The Yes Code www.carollook.com

Annual Tapping World Summit, Turning Possibilities into Realities, Mary Morrissey, www.MaryMorrissey.com

8ᵗʰ Annual Tapping World Summit, www.thetappingsolution.com, Mary Ayres, www.Tappingintoaction.com

Rich Dad Poor Dad, Rich Dad's Cashflow Quadrant: Rich Dad's Guide to Financial Freedom, Robert Kiyosaki http://www.richdad.com/

* You Are the Placebo, Breaking the Habit of Being Yourself: How to Lose Your Mind and Create a New One, Dr. Joe Dispenza http://www.drjoedispenza.com/

The Little Book of Gratitude: Create a life of happiness and wellbeing by giving thanks, Dr. Robert A. Emmons http://www.happinessandwellbeing.org/robert-emmons/

Bleed for This, based on the true story of Vinny Pazienza, Ben Younger, www.vinnypaz.com, *https://www.facebook.com/bleedforthis/*

About the Author

Hi There!

As I join you in your quest to Live Your Full Life, I feel it is essential that you get to know me.

My name is Deborah Lucero. ·

I am a wife and mother with a genuine devotion to share my story of hope, healing, and peace.

You may have seen me in my Thursday Inspirations Facebook Live Events. My journey began by helping others who have fibromyalgia, sharing techniques learned to honor the mind, body, soul, and spirit.

I've seen both sides. I went from being drugged up, asleep on my couch, taking 18 prescription medications a day to only taking all-natural vitamins and supplements. I was diagnosed with fibromyalgia and several other related medical conditions in July of 2013. Now all I need is all-natural vitamins/supplements, meditation, and exercise!

I have to admit I haven't always made the right choices. I didn't do it the easy way. I ignored my body. I tormented my mind with negative thoughts. I hated my life and who I had become. I shamed my spirit by not realizing that I needed to nurture myself.

My quest to transform my body, mind, soul, and spirit was rough, but now I understand the challenges, so I can help you succeed!

I have become a better person who is in love with life.

A Bit More About Me…

Many of you know, I am a certified occupational therapy assistant (COTA, retired) as well as a certified level 1 handwriting specialist and a certified infant/touch massage instructor.

Even though I had an education, it didn't teach me the steps on how to live a full life! I didn't get this basic message from anything I was taught in school or even in college. It was not something I learned in the workforce. This message wasn't there!

Sure, there were guidelines for exercise and a healthy diet. But what about my soul? What about my spirit? What about my mind, my thoughts, and my feelings? What about my emotions and all of those events that kept me frozen in time? That prevented me from realizing I am an amazing being or I am worthy of health, wealth, love, and happiness?

My life was a mess! To make a long story short, I did not practice proper self-care at any point in my life. I also did not have coping skills to process and release emotions not serving me. After the loss of my father when I was 23, I stuffed my feelings down. I again found myself grief-stricken after losing my maternal grandmother, my rock, in 2012. I was sick and tired after being diagnosed with multiple medical conditions starting that same year. I felt broken after a car accident in 2014. I felt stuck, limited, and disgusted with my financial situation and personal relationships.

As I immersed myself in the personal growth and self-development field, I realized that I was doing things all wrong! I needed to embrace my body, forgive my mind, love my soul, and honor my spirit! So, I began to nurture myself at every level to slowly heal. I noticed that these positive changes were improving all areas of my life. I kept up these new healthy habits which allowed me to make a permanent difference.

After I cleaned up my lifestyle, I had so many people ask me how I did it. I also realized there are many people living unfulfilled lives. So, I was inspired to create my 5-Step Process which includes Detox, Releasing Emotion, Mindset, Reprogramming Your Mind, and Exercise/Physical Activity. It is the foundation of my Healing Insights 70-Day Course and The 5-Step Process For Fibromyalgia Relief. I also developed The Wellness Plan, a monthly subscription plan to maintain lasting change, to apply the 5- Steps to daily life. I have written a book titled *BE F*#%ING AMAZING! 70 Healing Insights to Live Your Full Life* which will be available in 2018!

I am here to help you realize you are worthy! With my guidance and support, you will learn to nurture your Mind, Body, Soul, and Spirit! So you can Live Your Full Life! You can reach your full potential!

My goal is to help you discover how to use the Power of the Mind, Positive Thoughts, and Abundant Mindset to improve all areas of your life. Together we can spread the word of hope, healing, and peace!

Thank you and I can't wait to see you in the 70-Day Course!

Printed in the United States
By Bookmasters